HISTOLOGY
Laboratory Manual

AF530674

HISTOLOGY Laboratory Manual

Sayee Rajangam
Ex-Professor
Department of Anatomy
International Medical School
Bengaluru, Karnataka, India

Leelavathy N
Ex-Associate Professor
Department of Anatomy
International Medical School
Bengaluru, Karnataka, India

RN Kulkarni
Ex-Professor and Head
Department of Anatomy
International Medical School
Bengaluru, Karnataka, India

Foreword
Flossie Jayakaran

JAYPEE *The Health Sciences Publisher*
New Delhi | London | Panama

Jaypee Brothers Medical Publishers (P) Ltd.

Headquarters
Jaypee Brothers Medical Publishers (P) Ltd.
4838/24, Ansari Road, Daryaganj
New Delhi 110 002, India
Phone: +91-11-43574357
Fax: +91-11-43574314
E-mail: jaypee@jaypeebrothers.com

Overseas Offices
J.P. Medical Ltd.
83, Victoria Street, London
SW1H 0HW (UK)
Phone: +44-20 3170 8910
Fax: +44(0) 20 3008 6180
E-mail: info@jpmedpub.com

Jaypee Brothers Medical Publishers (P) Ltd.
17/1-B, Babar Road, Block-B, Shaymali
Mohammadpur, Dhaka-1207
Bangladesh
Mobile: +08801912003485
E-mail: jaypeedhaka@gmail.com

Jaypee-Highlights Medical Publishers Inc.
City of Knowledge, Bld. 235, 2nd Floor, Clayton
Panama City, Panama
Phone: +1 507-301-0496
Fax: +1 507-301-0499
E-mail: cservice@jphmedical.com

Jaypee Brothers Medical Publishers (P) Ltd.
Bhotahity, Kathmandu, Nepal
Phone: +977-9741283608
E-mail: kathmandu@jaypeebrothers.com

Website: www.jaypeebrothers.com
Website: www.jaypeedigital.com

Inquiries for bulk sales may be solicited at: jaypee@jaypeebrothers.com

Histology: Laboratory Manual

First Edition: **2017**

ISBN: 978-93-86150-94-3

Printed at: Samrat Offset Pvt. Ltd.

Dedicated to

Our Teachers, Students and Family

Foreword

I have great pleasure in writing the foreword *Histology: Laboratory Manual* on the study of histology of the human tissues. This has been based on the general and systemic study of the body tissues.

I have perused the notes and the contents in the form of microphotographs and tables, and found that this is a very apt book for medical students. The study material is presented in an easy-to-read format. I noted that the illustrations are microphotographs of actual student slides, and are labeled profusely to facilitate recognition of the tissues in the normal systems.

Great care has been taken to demonstrate all the tissues under scanner, low power of the microscope as well as under the high power. Recognition is facilitated by labeling and drawing attention to the arrangement. The details are beautifully classified, demonstrating how structure decides the functioning of the cells and tissues. Embryological origins are indicated to logically show how origins dictate functions.

The notes are brief, and outline the layers in the wall of hollow organs or their arrangements in solid organs, the function of each layer, and how the same tissue is arranged in different locations of a system. Each set of microphotographs and subject matter is followed by tabular columns that facilitate learning using keywords and concepts. This is of great help to all medical students, who have to cope with the English medium of instructions, and also have to learn innumerable technical terms in a very short time.

I have known the authors—Professor Sayee Rajangam, Dr RN Kulkarni and Dr Leelavathy N, for many years as colleagues and friends. I am impressed by the work they have put in using all their years of experience in teaching, to help students to learn this subject. I wish them and the students who will find this book invaluable, all the best as they learn and use this information throughout their medical career.

Flossie Jayakaran
Ex-Professor
Department of Anatomy
International Medical School
Bengaluru, Karnataka, India

Preface

It is the wish of each teacher to bring forth his/her knowledge and experience in a teaching manual. The task is performed in coordination with the syllabus, curriculum and with the advent in the technology.

Global education is the term in vogue. Hence, in the 'user-friendly' *Histology: Laboratory Manual*, comprehensive basic information is provided to the undergraduates in the faculty of Medicine.

The histological pictures were captured, computerized and labeled from the slides that were demonstrated at the time of practical sessions in histology.

It is to be noted that the manual is facilitatory to the drawings to be drawn by the students in the record books in histology.

It is hoped that the configuration of the *Histology: Laboratory Manual* has coordinated the cognitive (theory), affirmative (communication) and practical (drawing/labeling) skills in the teaching and learning processes of histology in anatomy.

Sayee Rajangam
Leelavathy N
RN Kulkarni

Acknowledgments

The Associate Dean Professor, Dr Sudha Suresh, International Medical School, Bengaluru, Karnataka, India, and Gokula Education Foundation, Bengaluru are acknowledged for their encouragement.

Grateful thanks to our teachers for their guidance, and colleagues and students for their suggestions.

M/s Jaypee Brothers Medical Publishers (P) Ltd, New Delhi, India, is thanked for the publication of *Histology: Laboratory Manual*.

We thank our family for their support.

Contents

CHAPTER

1

Microscope

The basic parts of the light microscope (Fig. 1.1) are the frame, illuminating and magnifying systems.

FRAME

- Base supports the microscope.
- Arm has knobs for coarse and fine adjustments; arm is lifted in the transport of the microscope.
- Stage is for placing the slide containing the object and could be moved up and down.
- Body tube houses the optical system.

ILLUMINATING SYSTEM

- Mirror (concave/plain) reflects the external light to illuminate the object.
- Condenser brings the parallel light to focus in a narrow area and when the microscope is fully raised, it brightly illuminates the object.
- Iris diaphragm should be adjusted in such a way, that it permits the control of the light beam, so as to attain the best contrast of the specimen, i.e. the object and maximum resolving power of the objective.

MAGNIFYING SYSTEM

- Objectives (scanner/low power/high power/oil immersion) are for the initial magnification of the specimen and for producing the primary magnified image of the specimen.
- Eyepiece increases the magnification of the primary image formed by the objective.

TOTAL MAGNIFICATION

- Magnification of the eyepiece X objective.

For example, the inscriptions on the eyepiece and on low power objective are X10, then, the magnification is 100.

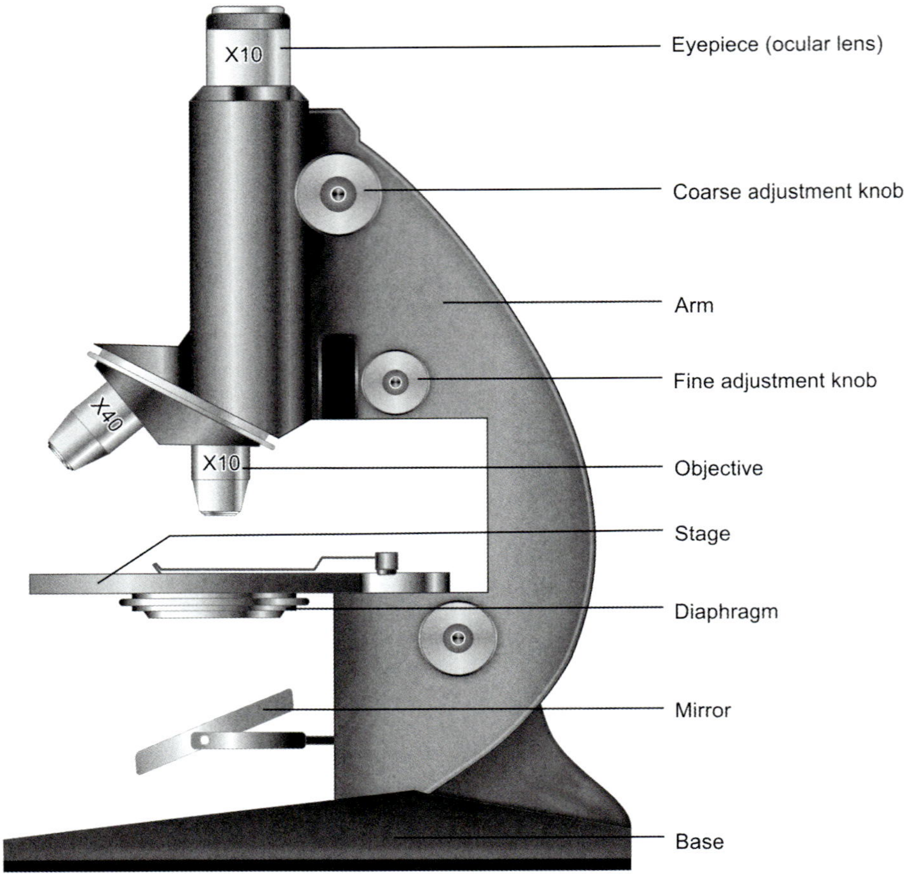

FIGURE 1.1 Microscope

CHAPTER

2

The Cell

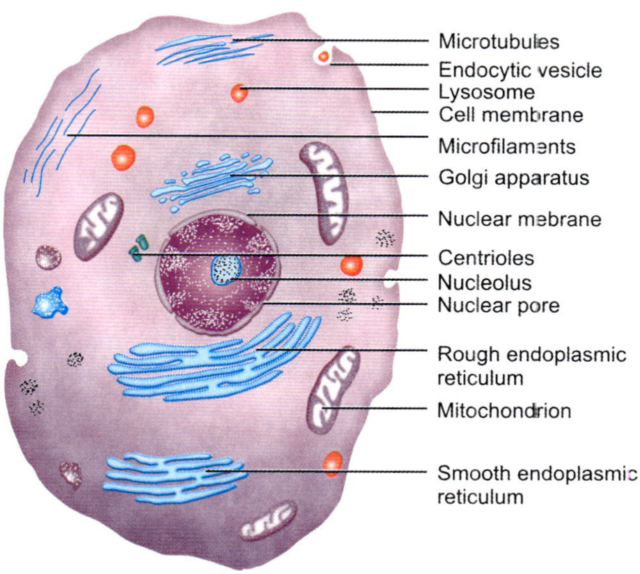

FIGURE 2.1 The cell

- Cells, the structural and functional units of the body, vary greatly in size, shape and structure and are adaptive for different functions.
- Cells surrounded by the cell membrane, consist of nucleus, cytoplasm and organelles (Fig. 2.1).
- Cytoplasm inside the cell has cytosol, a gel-like fluid and the organelles of the cell.
- Organelles (nucleus, endoplasmic reticulum, Golgi apparatus, mitochondria, lysosomes) perform the functions of the cell.
- Nucleus contains the genetic material and also controls the cell activities.
- Tissues (epithelial/connective/muscle, nerve) are the cells with similar morphology and function; specific tissues form the organs (stomach, brain, bladder); the integrated tissues and organs constitute the functional systems (urogenital/nervous).

CHAPTER

3

Epithelial Tissue

- Epithelial tissue is comprised of uninterrupted layers of cells and covers nearly all the external and internal surfaces of the body.
- Epithelium is the derivative of ectoderm, mesoderm and endoderm.
- Epithelial cells are mostly classified by the shape, the layers, i.e. stratification and the specializations on the surface (cilia/microvilli).
- Cells resting on basement membrane are tightly linked to each other.
- Cells polar in nature have apical and basal parts.
- Cells are avascular, but have high regenerative capacity.

SHAPE

- *Squamous*: Thin and flat
- *Cuboidal*: Short cylinders, but from the side appears like cubes
- *Columnar:* Looks like columns or cylinders.

STRATIFICATION

- *Simple*: One layer of cells
- *Stratified*: Two or more layers, one stacked above the basement layer
- *Pseudostratified*: One layer, but irregular lengths.

SPECIALIZATIONS

- Keratinized cells contain the protein, keratin
- Ciliated cells have the cilia.

Types	*Simple squamous epithelium (Fig. 3.1A)*	*Simple cuboidal epithelium (Fig. 3.1B)*	*Simple columnar epithelium (Fig. 3.1C)*
Cells	• One cell layer • All cells rest on the basement membrane • Width and depth of the cells greater than the height • Pavement epithelium • Regular hexagonal pattern	• One cell layer • All cells rest on the basement membrane • Cells cuboidal in shape • Width, depth and height are of the same dimensions	• One cell layer • All cells rest on the basement membrane • Height of the cells more than the depth and width
Nuclei	Flat or round or oval in shape, central in position	Centrally placed spherical nuclei	Oval elongated nuclei, towards the base of the cells
Function	Diffusion of gas or fluid	Absorption, excretion secretion	Absorption, secretion
Example	Mesothelium (peritoneal, pleural and pericardial cavities), Endothelium (heart, blood and lymph vessels), alveoli of lung	Collecting tubules of kidney, small excretory ducts of salivary glands and pancreas	Stomach, small intestine, gallbladder

Types	*Pseudostratified ciliated columnar epithelium/respiratory epithelium (Fig. 3.1D)*	*Transitional epithelium/urothelium (Fig. 3.1G)*
Cells	• Single layer of cells with cilia • All cells rest on the basement membrane, but short cells do not extend to the lumen	In the relaxed state, cells in the • Deep layers, cuboidal • Intermediate layers, polygonal • Superficial layers, large umbrella shaped cells In the stretched state, cells in the intermediate and surface layers, flattened
Nuclei	At different levels	Round or oval Cells may be multinucleated and covered by glycocalyx
Function	Propulsion of the mucus and the trapped particles to the pharynx	Accommodation of stretch and withstanding the toxicity of the urine
Example	Trachea	Ureter, urinary bladder

Types	*Stratified squamous nonkeratinized epithelium (Fig. 3.1E)*	*Stratified squamous keratinized epithelium (Fig. 3.1F)*
Cells	2 or more cell layers, only the basal cells rest on the basement membrane Cells in the • Deep layers, cuboidal or columnar • Intermediate layers, polyhedral • Superficial layers, squamous	Structure same as in the stratified squamous nonkeratinized epithelium, except for the superficial cells consisting of the protein keratin, dead and fibrous
Nuclei	All cells are nucleated	All cells, except the cells in the superficial layers, nucleated
Function	Withstanding the abrasion	Withstanding the abrasion and dessication
Example	Esophagus	Thick skin

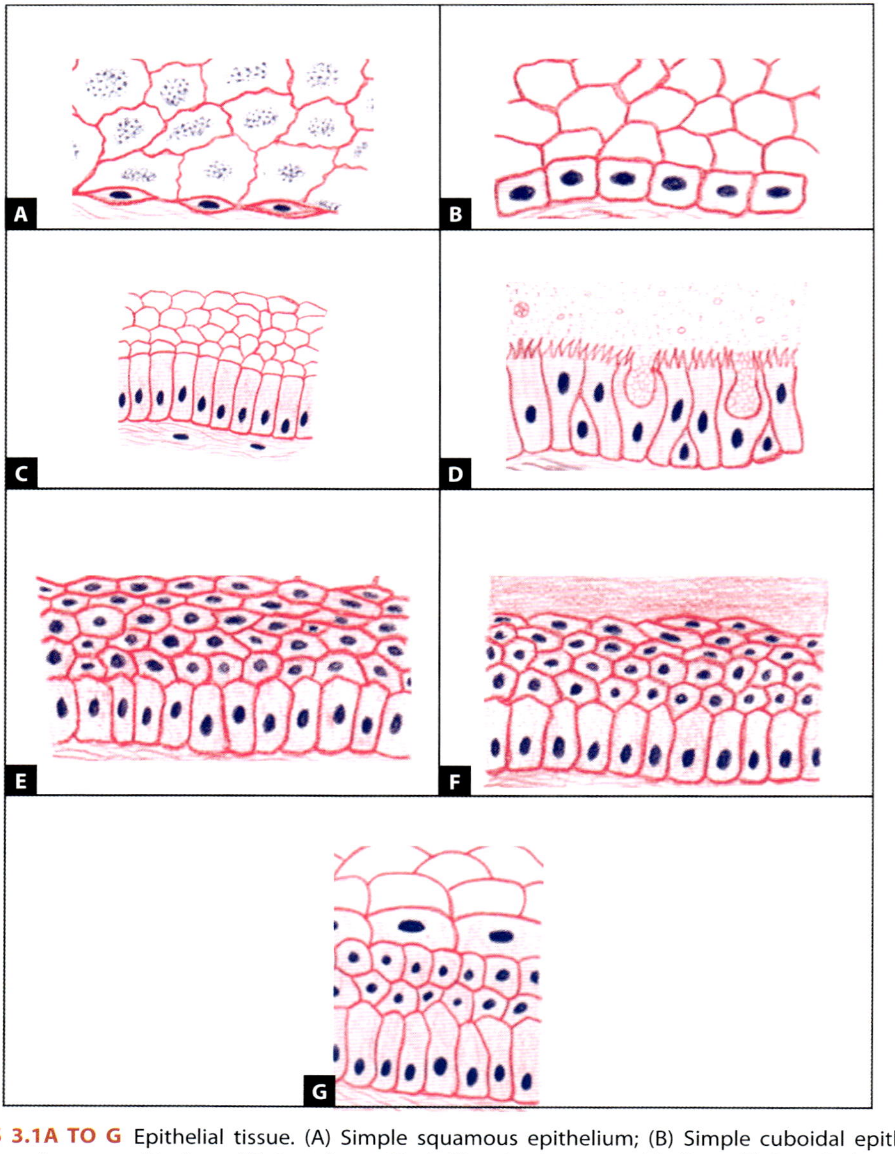

FIGURES 3.1A TO G Epithelial tissue. (A) Simple squamous epithelium; (B) Simple cuboidal epithelium; (C) Simple columnar epithelium; (D) Pseudostratified ciliated columnar epithelium; (E) Stratified squamous nonkeratinized epithelium; (F) Stratified squamous keratinized epithelium; (G) Transitional epithelium (urothelium)

CHAPTER

4

Connective Tissue

INTRODUCTION

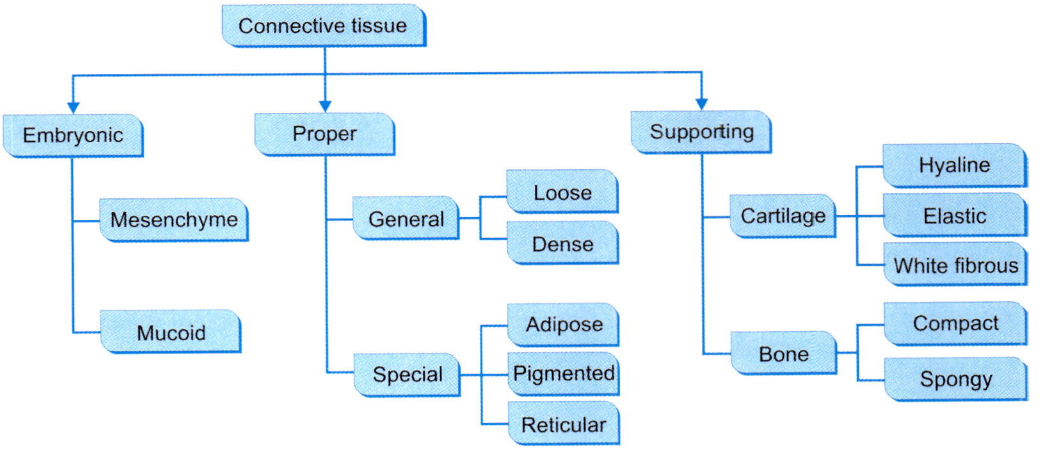

Mostly of mesodermal origin and provides support.

- Major constituents are the cells and the extracellular matrix (fibers and ground substance). Ground substance consists mainly three groups:
  1. Glycosaminoglycans (GAGs or mucopolysaccharides)
  2. Proteoglycans
  3. Glycoproteins
- Cells are the fibroblasts (synthesis and maintenance of extracellular matrix), macrophages (tissue scavengers and immune function), mast cells (secretion of histamine), plasma cells (formation of antibody), mesenchymal cells (stem cells), lymphocytes (defense and immune function) and adipose cells (storage and metabolism of fat).
- Fibers are the collagen, reticular and elastic fibers.
- Found throughout the body as the packing material and for binding the skin, membranes, vessels, nerves, muscles and also for binding any other tissues together.

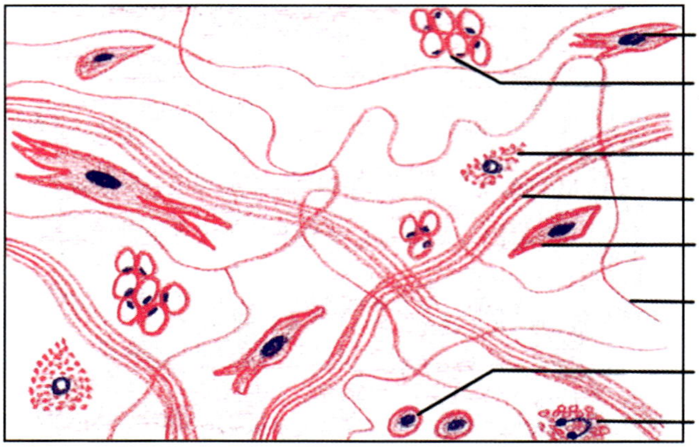

FIGURE 4.1 Loose areolar connective tissue, hematoxylin and eosin (H & E), X40

LOOSE CONNECTIVE TISSUE (FIG. 4.1)

- Consists of an extensive network of fibers, secreted by the cells of connective tissue, the fibroblasts.
- Collagen fibers, thicker and light-stained are the most numerous.
- Elastic fibers, thinner and dark-stained are also seen.
- Other connective tissue cells are present.

CARTILAGE

Cartilage a special form of supporting connective tissue is composed of cells (chondrocytes) and extracellular matrix (ground substance and fibers). More than 95% of cartilage consists of extracellular matrix, that is solid and firm, but allows flexibility and resilient to compression. Cartilage is mostly avascular and the exchange of the metabolites is through diffusion.

Based on the density and types of fibers in the extracellular matrix, cartilage is classified into three types:

1. Hyaline
2. Elastic
3. White fibrous.

Hyaline Cartilage

Hyaline cartilage, the most common cartilage has few collagen fibers and aggregations of chondrocytes in lacunae embedded in the amorphous matrix. Because of the similar refractive index, to both the ground substance and the fibers, the matrix is amorphous (glassy/transparent/homogeneous). Matrix contains type II collagen appearing as network of fine fibrils. Chondrocytes synthesizes the ground substance and the fibers of the cartilage. In embryos, hyaline cartilage serves as the model for most of the bones. In general, the process of the calcification is not seen in the hyaline cartilage.

Section under scanner (Fig. 4.2) shows the blue color stained matrix; throughout which ovoid spaces, the lacunae are distributed. Lacunae are the light and unstained spaces containing the

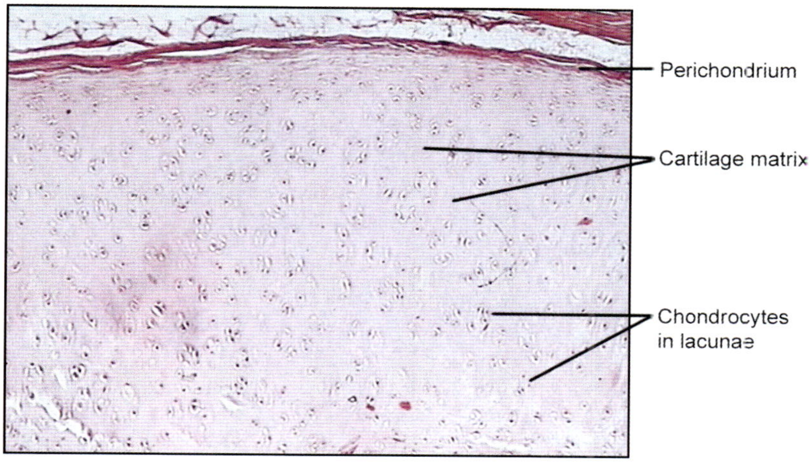

FIGURE 4.2 Hyaline cartilage, H & E, X40

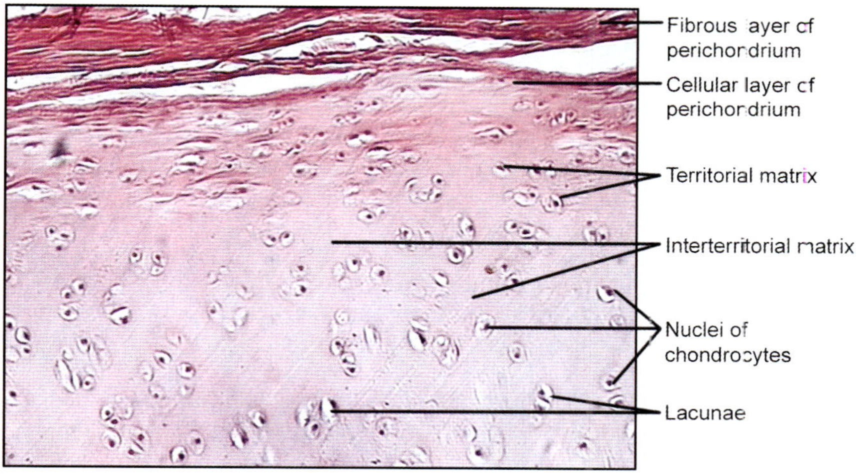

FIGURE 4.3 Hyaline cartilage, H & E, X100

cartilage cells, the chondrocytes. Cartilage is covered by perichondrium, which serves as the source to the formation of the new cartilage.

Section under low power (Fig. 4.3) shows the two distinctive layers of perichondrium; an outer fibrous layer and an inner cellular chondrogenic layer. Collagen fibers are masked by the ground substance and hence are not seen. The other component, sulfated glycosaminoglycans exhibit basophilia with hematoxylin stain.

Thin matrix separates the two or more chondrocytes in the lacunae located close to each other. Single parental chondroblast give rise to the group of chondrocytes. The mature cells

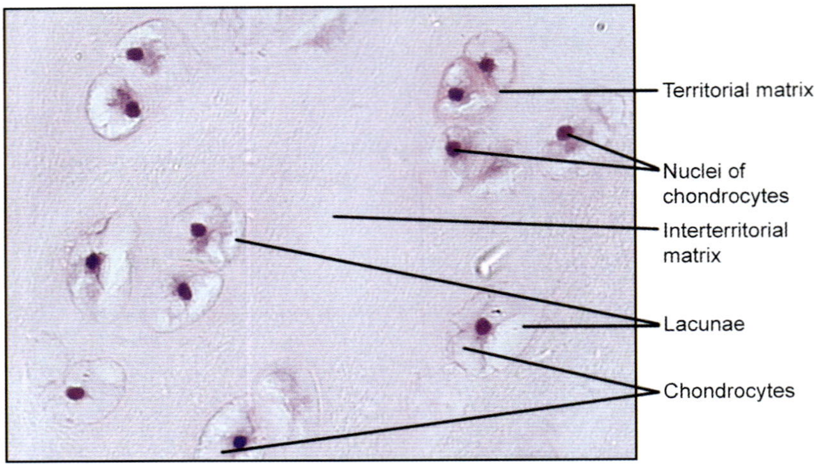

FIGURE 4.4 Hyaline cartilage, H & E, X400

(chondrocytes) are seen towards the center as isogenous groups (cell nests/clusters) and immature cells (chondroblasts) towards the periphery are usually present in single numbers.

Section under high power (Fig. 4.4) shows the matrix immediately surrounding the lacunae; more deeply stained regions form the territorial matrix and the light-stained matrix between the chondrocytes form the interterritorial matrix. Each chondrocyte has granular cytoplasm and nucleus. During histology preparations, the cells shrink and the lacunae appear as clear spaces.

Elastic Cartilage

Elastic cartilage has matrix containing a number of bundles of branched elastic fibers and elastic lamellae. Collagen is also the constituent of the matrix and is seen in the perichondrium. The elastic material imparts properties of elasticity. Cartilage is surrounded by perichondrium and normally does not calcify.

Section under scanner (Fig. 4.5) shows the blue color stained matrix and the unstained lacunae with chondrocytes. Cartilage is covered by the perichondrium and the two layers of the perichondrium are appreciable.

Section under low power (Fig. 4.6) shows the deep pink stained elastic fibers entering the cartilage matrix from the surrounding perichondrium and distributed throughout as the branching and anastomosing fibers of various sizes. The density of the fibers varies among the elastic cartilages as well as among the different areas of the same cartilage and are more evident in the periphery.

Some lacunae are arranged in pairs separated by a thin plate of matrix indicate that the cells are divided from the same parent cell. As the cells move away from each other, the cells secrete a plate of cartilage matrix. Larger chondrocytes in lacunae are more prevalent in the interior of the cartilage. The smaller and flatter chondrocytes are located peripherally in the inner chondrogenic layer of the perichondrium.

Section under high power (Fig. 4.7) shows elastic fibers as elongate profiles. Most chondrocytes occupy only part of the lacunae, due to shrinkage and also due to the fact that the large lipid droplets

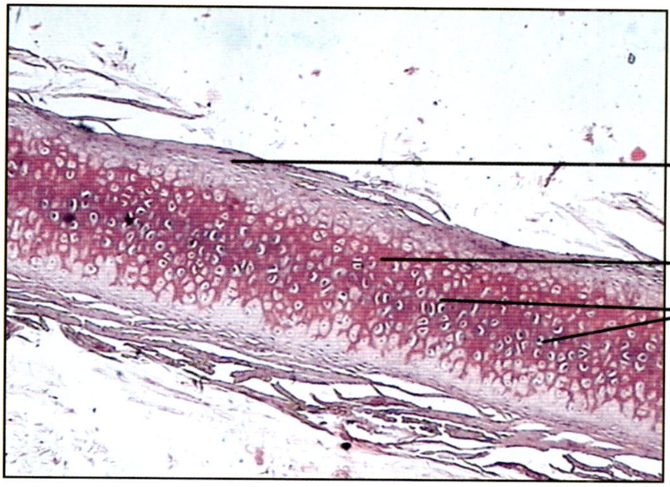

FIGURE 4.5 Elastic cartilage, H & E, X40

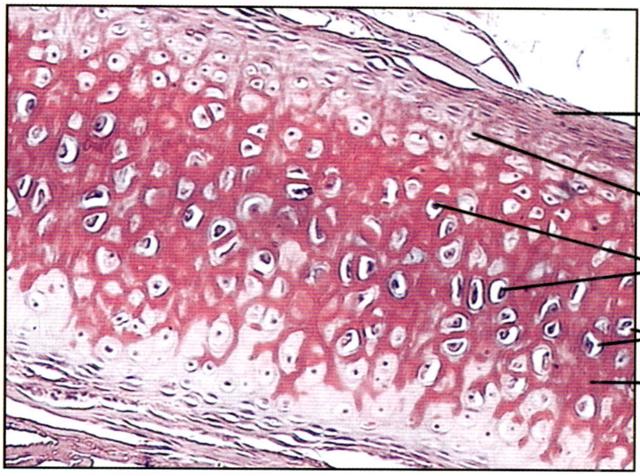

FIGURE 4.6 Elastic cartilage, H & E, X100

in the older chondrocytes are lost during the processing of the tissue. Hence, lacunae stand out as the light, unstained areas against the darkly stained matrix.

Fibrous Cartilage

Fibrous cartilage is characterized by hyaline cartilage matrix alternating with abundant and thick layers of type I and II dense collagen fibers. Chondrocytes are usually distributed in rows.

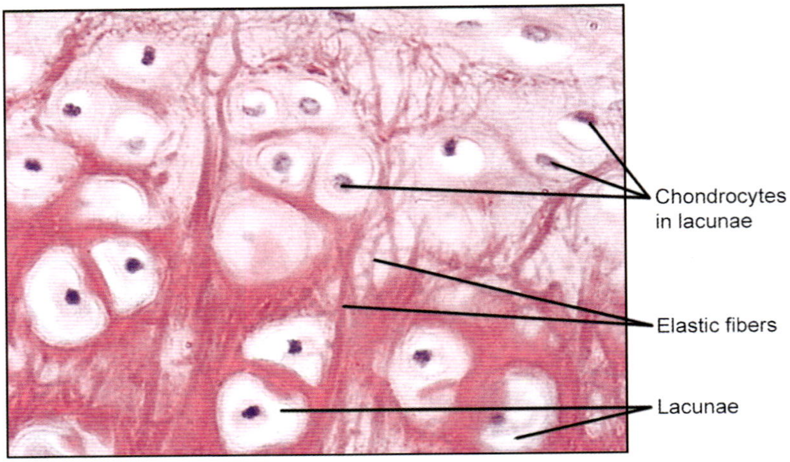

FIGURE 4.7 Elastic cartilage, H & E, X400

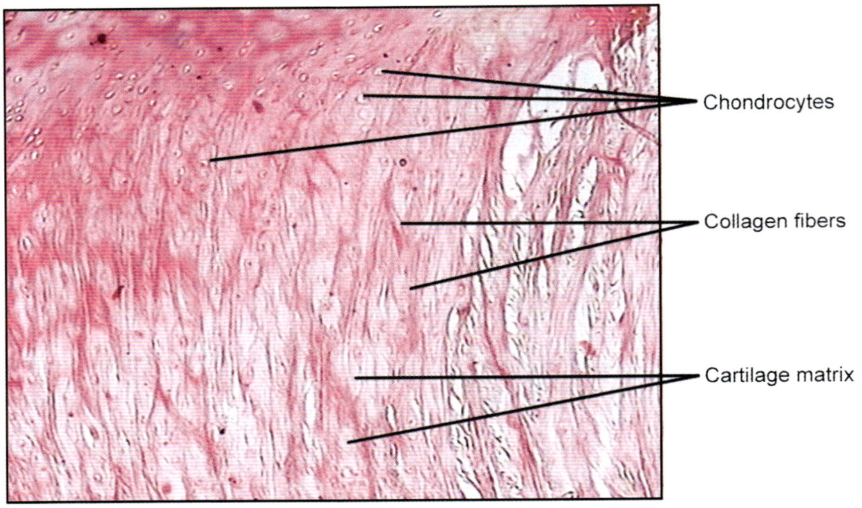

FIGURE 4.8 Fibrous cartilage, H & E, X40

The presence of the fibrous cartilage is associated with sites where resilience is required, as in dense connective tissue to help to absorb the sudden physical impact where resistance to both compressive and shearing forces is required.

Perichondrium is absent, because, fibrous cartilage usually forms transitional area between hyaline cartilage and tendon or ligament.

Section under scanner (Fig. 4.8) shows the collagen fibers in bundles stained dark pink alternating with the light stained matrix. The amount of the cartilage varies, as seen in the picture.

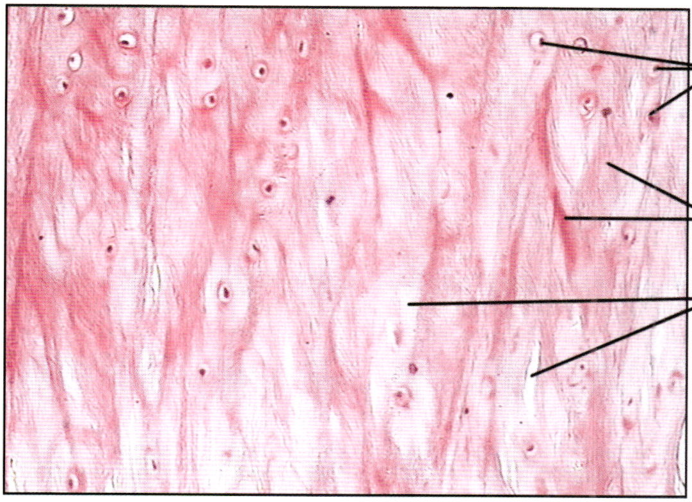

FIGURE 4.9 Fibrous cartilage, H & E, X100

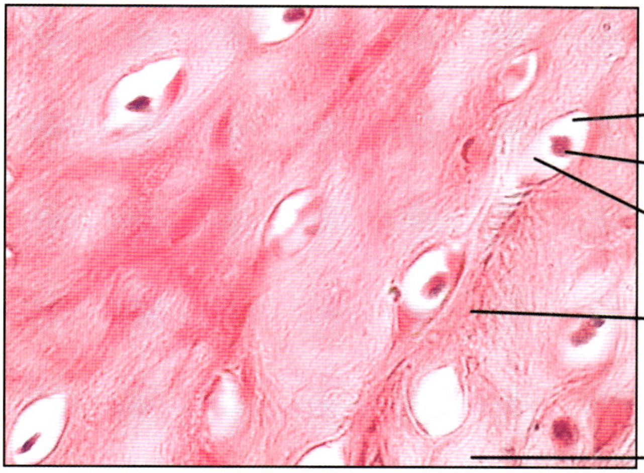

FIGURE 4.10 Fibrous cartilage, H & E, X400

The cartilage cells and the matrix occupy less portion of the tissue mass. Fibroblasts are few. Chondrocytes are present in rows, between the bundles of the collagen fibers in the matrix.

Section under low power (Fig. 4.9) shows the chondrocytes of similar size. Variation in size is not observed, as in hyaline or elastic cartilage. Chondrocytes are present in rows or in close spatial groups (isogenous groups).

The light stained homogeneous area around the lacunae is the cartilage matrix.

Section under high power (Fig. 4.10) shows the chondrocytes in rows within the lacunae, between the bundles of the collagen fibers in the matrix. The deep stained cytoplasm and nuclei of the chondrocytes are seen. Lacunae could be observed in some, because of the shrinkage of the cells.

POINTS TO REMEMBER

Types	*Hyaline*	*Elastic*	*Fibrous*
Extracellular matrix	Homogeneous because of same refractive index for both ground substance and collagen fibers type 2. Collagen fibers type 2 embedded in ground substance	Dense network of branching elastic fibers and collagen fibers type 2 embedded in ground substance	Type 1 collagen fibers embedded in ground substance. Alternating dense bundles of collagen fibers
Ground substance	Mostly, type 2 collagen fibers embedded in glycosaminoglycans	Elastic and collagen fibers embedded	Type 1 collagen fibers embedded
Perichondrium Fibrocyte and chondrogenic layers	Present Absent over the articular cartilage	Present	Absent
Example	Nasal septum, structural framework of larynx, trachea and bronchi, articular cartilage, costal cartilage, most of the fetal skeleton	Auricle of external ear, auditory tube, parts of the epiglottis, cuneiform and corniculate cartilages of larynx	Intervertebral disc, articular disc of the temporomandibular and sternoclavicular joints, pubis symphysis, grooves for insertion of tendons or ligaments, menisci of knee joint

BONE

Bone, a specialized hard type of connective tissue is characterized by a mineralized extracellular matrix. Calcium phosphate, in the form of hydroxyapatite crystals is deposited along the collagen fibrils and in the osteoid (collagenous extracellular matrix with type I collagen). Bone serves as a storage site for calcium and phosphate, which are released to the blood to maintain the homeostasis. Bone provides the rigid and supporting framework to the body and with the attached muscles facilitates the movements of the body.

- Composed of cells and matrix called, osteoid mineralized by calcium hydroxyapatite, which gives the rigidity and strength.
- Lamellae (fibers and calcified matrix organized into thin plates) the most characteristic features.

- Lacunae, space situated within or between the lamellae, contain bone cells (osteocytes). Cytoplasmic processes of osteocytes project into the canaliculi, thin spaces extending from the lacunae.

Cells

- Osteoblasts synthesize the osteoid and mediate the mineralization and are present in lines along the surfaces of the bone.
- Osteocytes mature inactive bone cells are enclosed within osteoid, necessary for nutrition and maintenance of the bone.
- Osteoclasts, the bone phagocytic cells are required for the turnover and the remodeling of the bone.

Macroscopic Structure

Two Types of Bone are Distinguished

Trabecular bone (cancellous/spongy/medullary): It consists of delicate bars and sheets of bone trabeculae, which branch and intersect to form sponge, like network. Trabecular bone is seen in the ends of the long bones or epiphyses. The spaces in the medullary bone occupied by bone marrow are involved in hematopoiesis.

Compact bone (cortex): It does not have any spaces or hollow areas in the bone matrix. Compact bone forms the thick-walled tube of the shaft or diaphysis of the long bones and surrounds the marrow or medullary cavity. A thin layer of compact bone also covers the epiphyses of the long bones.

Bone is covered by periosteum and endosteum. Endosteum lines the surface of the bone facing the marrow cavity. Periosteum, the dense fibrous layers receives the attachments of the muscles, tendons and ligaments. Both periosteum and endosteum possess the osteogenic potency. The cells of the periosteum are capable of converting into the osteoprogenitor cells and osteoblasts.

The Dried Bone is Ground to a Thin Section, Mounted without Staining and Observed under the Microscope

Bone-transverse Section

Section under scanner (Fig. 4.11) (cross section (CS) or the transverse section (TS)) shows the structural unit of the compact bone, the osteon (haversian system), circled in black line. Each osteon, a cylindrical structure has layers of concentric lamellae arranged around central canal (haversian canal), containing the blood vessels, connective tissue and cells lining the surface of the bone material. Small black spaces seen in the section are the lacunae; lacunae appear black, since the spaces are filled with air.

Section under low power (Fig. 4.12) shows the perforating canals (Volkmann's canals), through which blood vessels reach the haversian canals, from the marrow cavity. Volkmann's canals may also connect adjacent haversian canals. The difference between the Volkmann's canals and haversian canals is that Volkmann's canal passes through the lamellae, whereas haversian canals are surrounded by the lamellae. The osteocytes in the lacunae appear as 'tiny' brown specks.

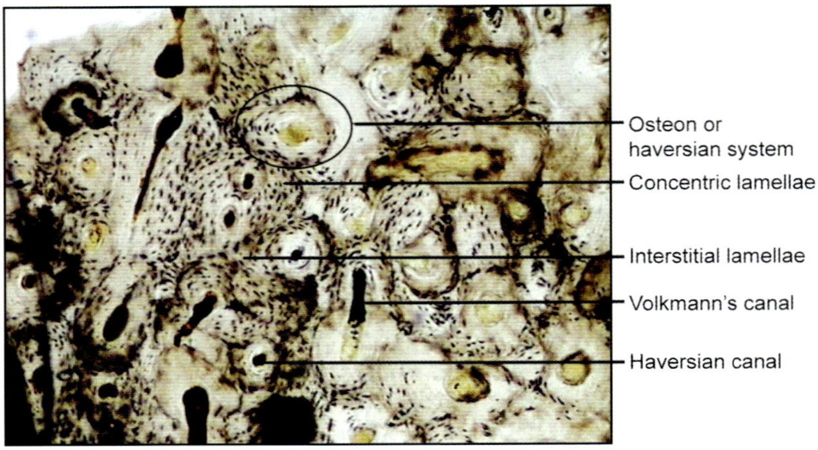

FIGURE 4.11 Bone, TS, Ground section, X40

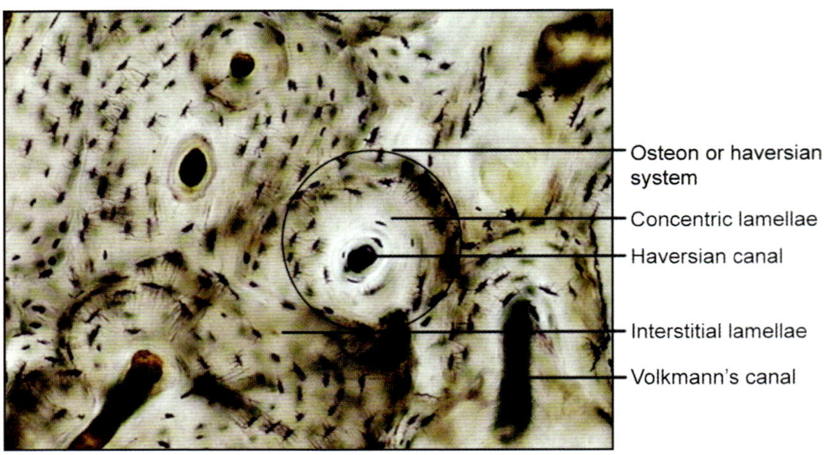

FIGURE 4.12 Bone, TS, Ground section, X100

Section under high power (Fig. 4.13) shows the canaliculi, radiating tiny canals (thread-like processes) from the lacunae in all directions. The canaliculi penetrate the lamellae and anastomose with the canaliculi of the other lacunae. In 'living bone' the processes of the osteocytes present in the lacunae intercommunicate with each other through the canaliculi.

Bone-longitudinal Section

Sections under scanner (X40) (Fig. 4.14) and low power (X100) (Fig. 4.15) show the ground dry bone in longitudinal plane, i.e. longitudinal section (LS). Haversian canal is coursing longitudinal and

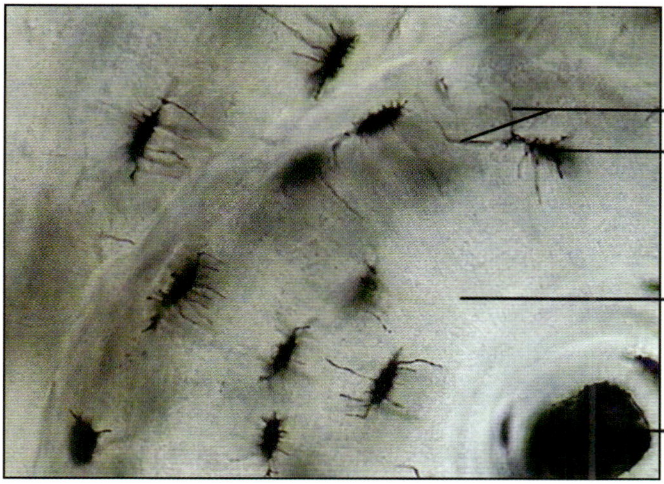

FIGURE 4.13 Bone, TS, Ground section, Osteon, X400

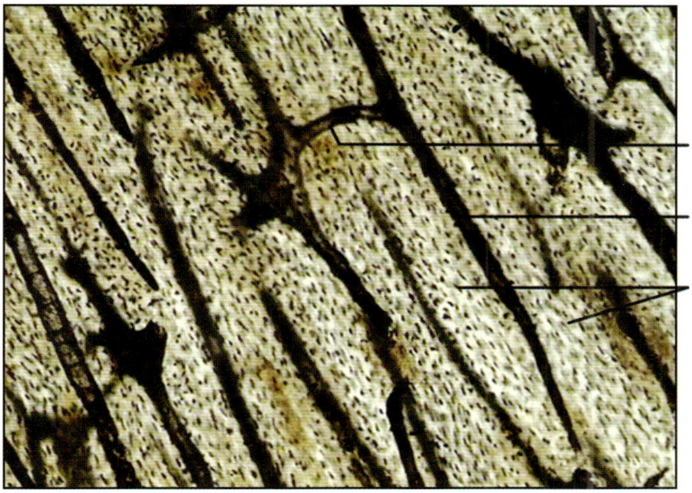

FIGURE 4.14 Bone, LS, Ground section, X40

seen as the vertical tube with branching. The lamellae, lacunae and radiating canaliculi run parallel to the haversian canal.

Also seen in the picture are the canals extending either in transverse or oblique direction, the perforating (Volkmann's) canals. Volkmann's canals join the adjacent haversian canals and also the marrow cavity and penetrate directly through the lamellae.

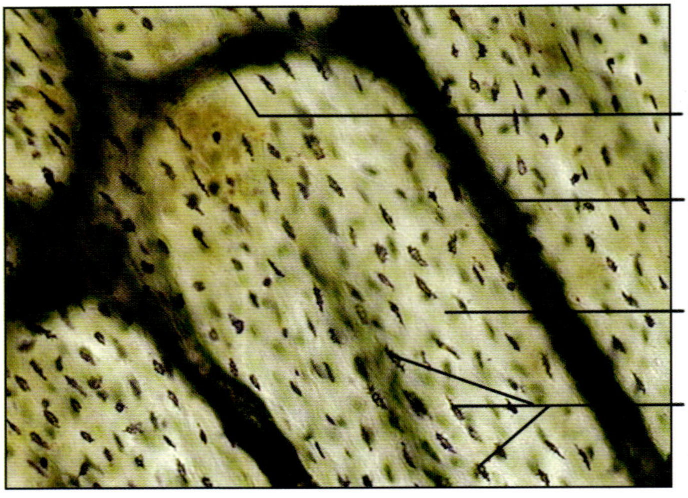

FIGURE 4.15 Bone, LS, Ground section, X100

POINTS TO REMEMBER

Bone: Transverse Section (TS)

- *Haversian system (osteon):* Haversian canal is surrounded by numerous concentric lamellae of bony matrix and concentric rings of flattened lacunae with or without osteocytes are seen.
- New and old haversian systems as well as interstitial haversian systems (former haversian systems) are present.
- Lamellae arranged at the periphery, near the marrow cavity and in between the osteons, constitute the outer circumferential lamellae, inner circumferential lamellae and interstitial lamellae.
- Canaliculi radiate from the lacunae are occupied with the processes of the osteocytes and the processes communicate with the processes from the other osteocytes, in the adjacent lamellae. The function of the canaliculi is for the circulation of the extracellular fluid and diffusion of the metabolites between the lacunae and vessels of haversian canals.
- Cement line is the thin modified matrix around the osteon.
- Bone is covered by the periosteum.

Bone: Longitudinal Section (LS)

- Longitudinal channels (haversian canals) are seen along with the oblique and transverse channels (Volkmann's canals) extending between the haversian canals and also endosteum communicate with each other.
- Lamellae are arranged parallel to the haversian canals.
- Lacunae with or without osteocytes are present.
- Periosteum is seen.

CHAPTER 5

Muscular Tissue

Muscular tissue is responsible for the movement of the body and its parts and for changing the size and shape of the internal organs. Muscular tissue is composed of cells having large amount of contractile proteins, the actin and myosin. Muscular tissue is classified depending on the appearance of the contractile proteins—striated and smooth muscle. Striated is further classified into skeletal and cardiac. Each type has structural and functional similarities as well as differences.

The cells of the muscular tissue are elongated, hence known as the fibers. The cytoplasm is known as the sarcoplasm and the cell membrane as sarcolemma. Each fiber contains numerous myofibrils containing actin and myosin arranged in a regular manner giving the characteristic feature of the cross-striated appearance in skeletal muscle and cardiac muscle. Skeletal muscle and cardiac muscle have blood supply; but, cardiac muscle even to the 'naked eye' appears brown, because of the rich blood supply. The innervation to the smooth muscle and cardiac muscle is from the autonomic nervous system (ANS); therefore, smooth and cardiac muscle are considered to be involuntary; whereas peripheral nervous system (PNS) supplies the skeletal muscle, also known as the voluntary muscle.

SMOOTH MUSCLE

Smooth muscle is found in viscera; i.e. in numerous organs belonging to the respiratory, digestive, urinary and genital systems. The protein filaments are not arranged in order and the muscle appears to be smooth or nonstriated. The smooth muscle fibers are involuntary. The smooth muscle fibers are small, spindle or fusiform shape with fine tapered ends and a single centrally situated nucleus. The size of the smooth muscle fibers may vary from blood vessel (20 μm) to small intestine (200 μm) and to 500 μm, during pregnancy in uterus. The adjacent smooth muscle cells are interconnected by gap junctions.

Section under scanner (Fig. 5.1) shows smooth muscle tissue (both TS and LS) and connective tissue (difficult to differentiate the light pink stained smooth muscle tissue and connective tissue).

Sections under low power (Fig. 5.2) and high power (Figs 5.3 and 5.4) show the fibers cut in LS and TS.

In TS, the smooth muscle cells and nuclei show different shapes and sizes because of the cut appearance in different plane and different place of the fibers. The section is through the center, then, the nucleus appears large and section is away from the center, nucleus may be seen as a small structure. In LS, smooth muscle fibers are spindle-shaped with tapered ends. The cytoplasm is darkly stained. The nucleus is ovoid or elongated.

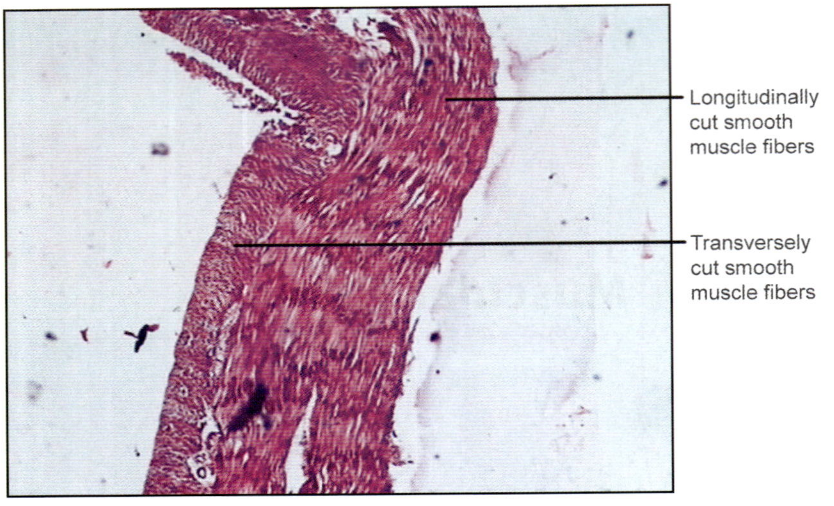

FIGURE 5.1 Smooth muscle, TS and LS, H & E, X40

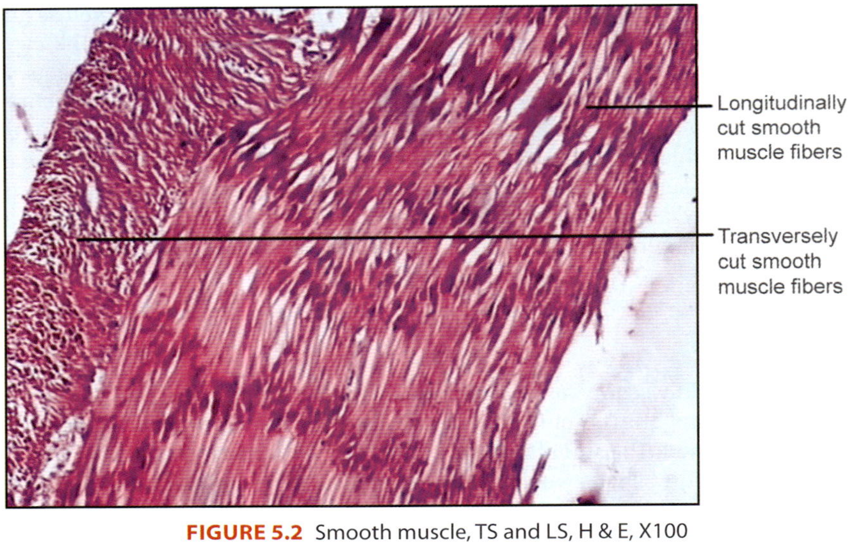

FIGURE 5.2 Smooth muscle, TS and LS, H & E, X100

SKELETAL MUSCLE

Skeletal muscle fibers are long, multinucleated cells with peripheral nuclei. Contractile filaments actin and myosin regularly arranged in the cytoplasm appear as cross-striations (light I band and dark A band).

The skeletal muscle is covered by dense, irregular connective tissue, the epimysium, from which a less dense irregular connective tissue extends inwards and divides into muscle bundles or

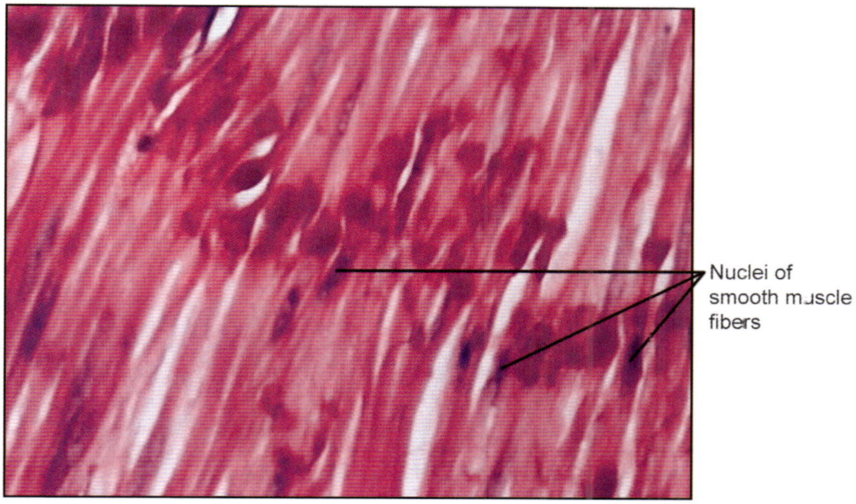

FIGURE 5.3 Smooth muscle, LS, H & E, X400

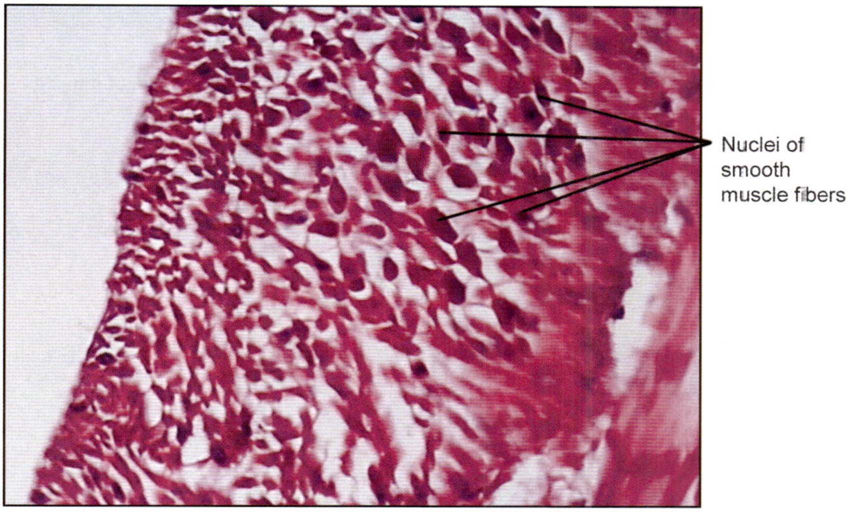

FIGURE 5.4 Smooth muscle, TS, H & E, X400

fascicles called perimysium. Individual muscle fibers are invested by a thin connective tissue called endomysium. Small blood vessels and capillaries are present in the connective tissue around each fiber.

Section under scanner (Fig. 5.5) shows both TS and LS of skeletal muscle. In TS, polygonal-shaped cells observed and in LS, the fibers are arranged parallel to each other.

Section under low power (Fig. 5.6) shows the fibers running parallel to each other and the multinuclei placed at periphery. Observe the air bubbles which could be mistaken for nuclei.

Section under high power (Fig. 5.7) shows the fibers with cross-striations and peripheral multinuclei. The two main bands A and I bands could be appreciated which are formed by

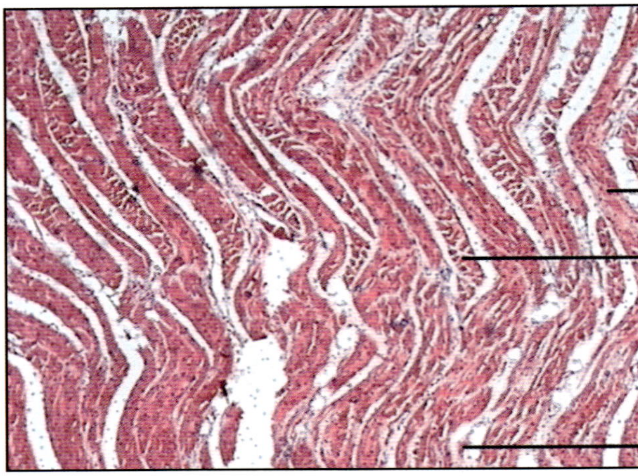

FIGURE 5.5 Skeletal muscle, TS and LS, H & E, X40

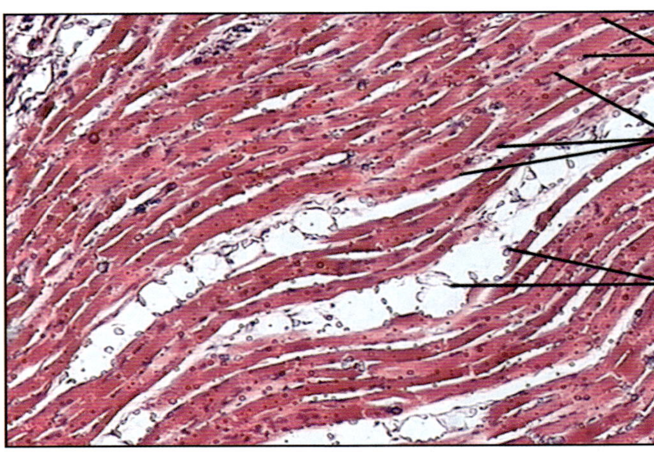

FIGURE 5.6 Skeletal muscle, LS, H & E, X100

myofilaments composed of contractile proteins myosin and actin. The A band, the dark band formed by the myosin filaments extend in the center and actin filaments extend at the sides. The myosin filaments not overlapped by actin filaments form the H band. The center of the H band is bisected by the M line. I band is the light band formed by the actin filaments attached to the Z line. The contractile apparatus extending between two adjacent Z lines is a sarcomere.

Cell membrane (sarcolemma) surrounds each fiber. Flat nuclei present just below the cell membrane are surrounded by the cytoplasm (sarcoplasm). Endomysium contains blood vessels, capillaries and fibrocytes. Cross-striations are identified as light stained I-bands and dark stained A-bands.

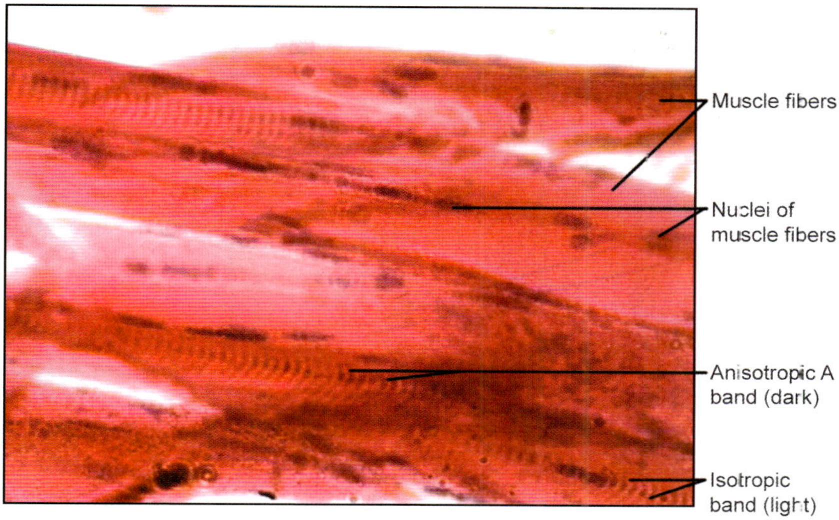

FIGURE 5.7 Skeletal muscle, LS, H & E, X400

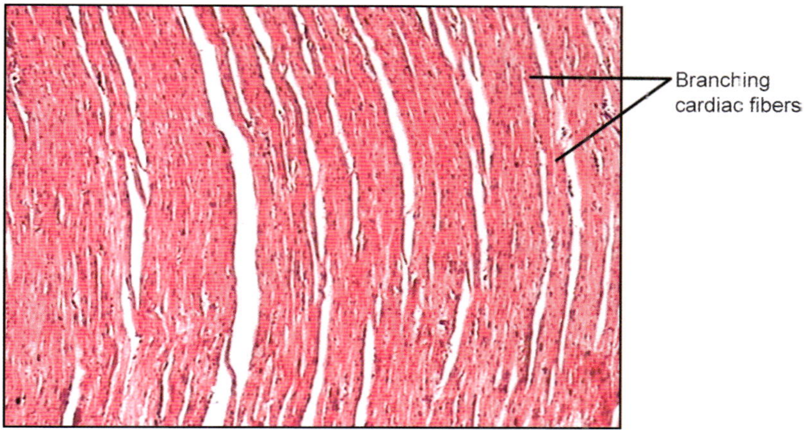

FIGURE 5.8 Cardiac muscle, H & E, X40

CARDIAC MUSCLE

Cardiac muscle is located in the walls and septa of heart and in the walls of large vessels that are attached to the heart. Cardiac muscle exhibits distinct cross-striations and small myofibrils in each fiber, as in skeletal muscle; but, it differs in other aspects. The individual cells are joined by complex junctions, the intercalated discs, so as to perform as a single functional unit. Each fiber has one nucleus, occasionally two nuclei in the center, unlike the skeletal muscle. The fibers are shorter than the skeletal muscle fibers and branched.

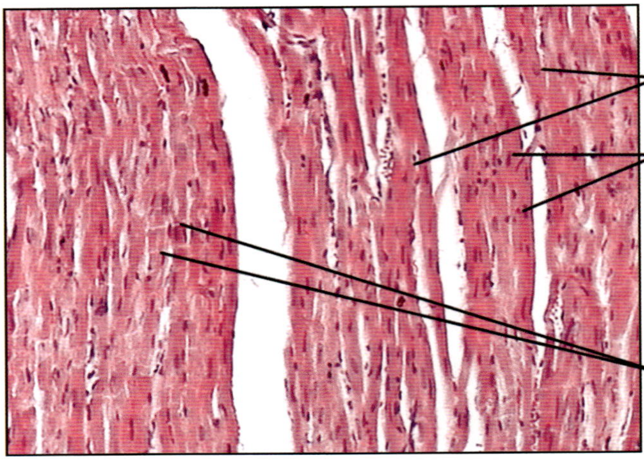

FIGURE 5.9 Cardiac muscle, H & E, X100

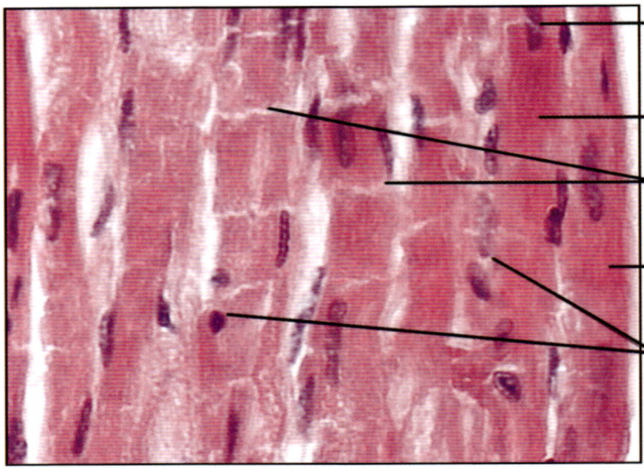

FIGURE 5.10 Cardiac muscle, H & E, X400

LS under scanner and low power (Figs 5.10 and 5.8) shows the fibers running parallel to each other and the branching from the fibers. The intercalated disc is not seen under scanner; under the low power seen, but not appreciated.

Section under high power (Fig. 5.9) shows, around the nuclei, the clear zones free of myofibrils and cross-striations, the perinuclear sarcoplasm. They contain cytoplasmic organelles not involved in the process of contraction. The characteristic feature is the intercalated disc; the dark stained structures found at the irregular intervals represent the specialized junctional complexes between adjacent cardiac muscle cells.

Intercalated discs functionally join adjacent cardiac muscle cells and rapidly spread the stimulus for contraction of the heart muscle. The diffusion of ions through the pores in gap junctions between individual cardiac muscle fibers coordinates the functions of the heart and allows the cardiac muscle to act as functional syncytium, thereby, allowing the stimuli for contraction to pass through the entire cardiac muscle.

POINTS TO REMEMBER

—	*Skeletal muscle*	*Cardiac muscle*	*Smooth muscle*
Muscle cells (fibers)	Long cylindrical unbranched muscle fibers	Tubular fibers branch and anastomoses	Spindle-shaped
Striations	• Cross-striations of alternating light (Isotropic or I bands) and dark bands (Anisotropic or A bands). • Light band bisected by a dark transverse line, the Z line. • Dark band shows the lighter zone in center, the H band.	Faint cross-striated banding patterns	Lack visible cross-striations
Nuclei	Multinucleated, flat or oval, peripherally arranged	Uninucleate, central in position	Uninucleate, central in position
Distinguishing feature	• Sarcomere, the smallest repetitive subunit of the contractile apparatus lies between two Z lines. • Sarcomere consists of thick (myosin) and thin (actin) filaments.	Intercalated disc, faintly seen, under the light microscope, represent the junctional complexes	—
Functions	Movements	Autonomic, rhythmic involuntary movements	Involuntary movement, i.e. churning of food, movement of urine from the kidney to the bladder, parturition of the fetus
Example	Muscles attached to the bone	Heart	Walls of hollow organs (stomach, intestine, uterus, ureter)

CHAPTER

6

Nerve Tissue

The components of the nervous system are the neurons, nerve fibers and neuroglia. Neurons are arranged as nuclei inside the CNS and as ganglia outside the CNS. Nerve fibers are the afferent (dendrites) and efferent (axons) fibers. Neuroglia are the Schwann cells and satellite cells in PNS and astrocytes, oligodendrocytes, microglia and ependymal cells in CNS.

Nervous system is divided into two parts the central nervous system (CNS) (brain and spinal cord) and the peripheral nervous system (PNS) (cranial and peripheral nerves, sympathetic and spinal ganglia). CNS and PNS deliver rapid and precise communication between the parts of the body.

PERIPHERAL NERVE

The peripheral nerve has numerous axons of various sizes surrounded by several layers of connective tissue, dividing the nerve into several bundles or fascicles. Outermost dense irregular connective tissue layer is the epineurium surrounding the whole nerve; around the fascicle is the thin connective tissue layer, the perineurium and around each fiber is the loose connective tissue layer of thin reticular fibers, the endoneurium.

TS under scanner (Fig. 6.1) shows several bundles or fascicles with accompanying blood vessels. Each fascicle is surrounded by perineurium that merges with the surrounding interfascicular connective tissue. Each individual nerve axon is surrounded by a delicate connective tissue layer, the endoneurium, which extends from the perineurium. Epineurium of the nerve is not seen.

Sections under the low (Fig. 6.2) and high (Fig. 6.3) power show a single nerve fascicle, where myelin sheaths surrounding the axons are seen as empty spaces. Numerous nuclei seen between the individual nerve axons represent the nuclei of the Schwann cells or neurolemmocytes. Schwann cells in PNS form the insulating, lipid rich myelin sheaths around the axons. Surrounding the myelin sheath (white space) is the connective tissue sheath called endoneurium.

DORSAL ROOT OR SPINAL GANGLION

Spinal ganglia are aggregations of neurons, outside CNS. Spinal ganglion is situated on the dorsal nerve root of spinal nerve. Most of the ganglia have round unipolar neurons and in between are the nerve fascicles representing the peripheral processes of the bifurcated single axon of the unipolar neuron. The axons do not have synaptic connections.

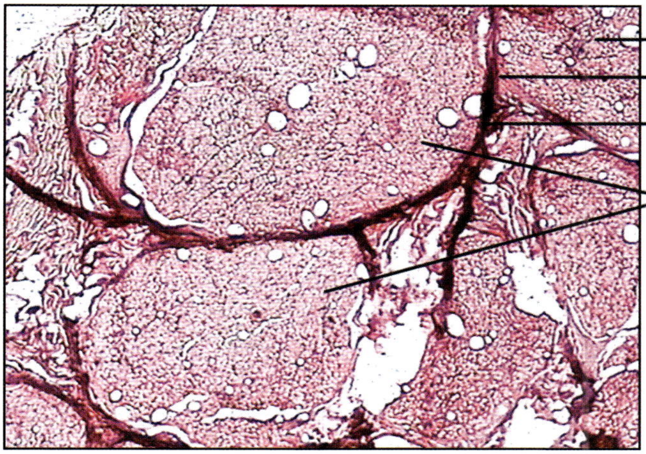

FIGURE 6.1 Peripheral nerve, TS, H & E, X40

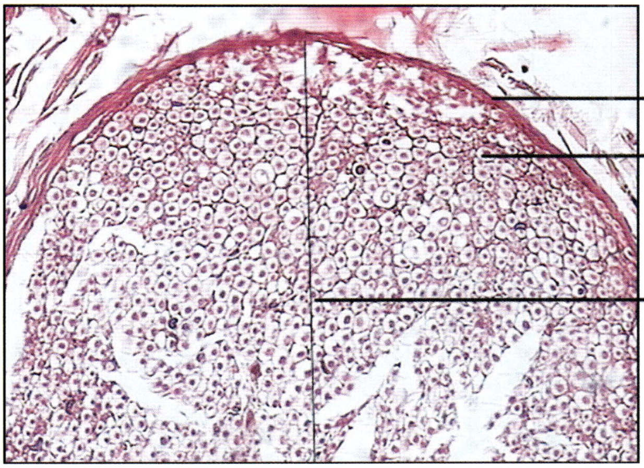

FIGURE 6.2 Peripheral nerve, TS, H & E, X100

Section under scanner shows (Fig. 6.4) the ganglion enclosed by an irregular connective tissue layer with adipose cells, nerves and blood vessels merging with the epineurium of spinal nerve. The dorsal and ventral roots unite to form the spinal nerve are not seen. The roots are surrounded by delicate connective tissue or the pia mater and arachnoid mater of the spinal cord. The ganglion neurons are arranged in groups. The bundles of nerve fibers run between the cell groups.

In low power, the section (Fig. 6.5) shows the ganglion neurons with the nuclei. The satellite cells are seen and identified well. The satellite cells are large, round and closely arranged to each other. Some neurons are seen without the nuclei; since the section has not passed through the center of the neurons. Some neurons contain small clumps of lipofuscin pigment in the cytoplasm.

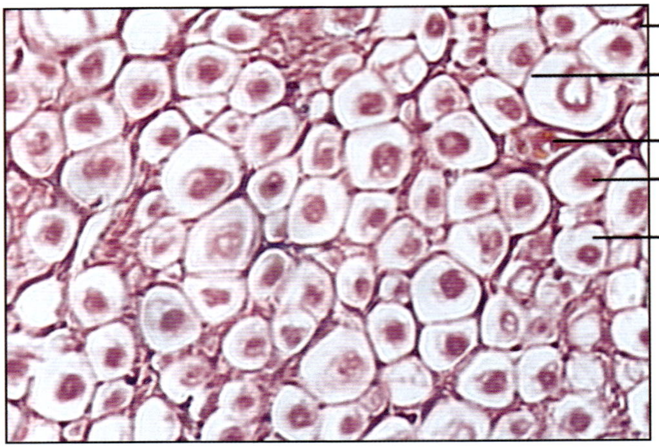

FIGURE 6.3 Peripheral nerve, TS, H & E, X400

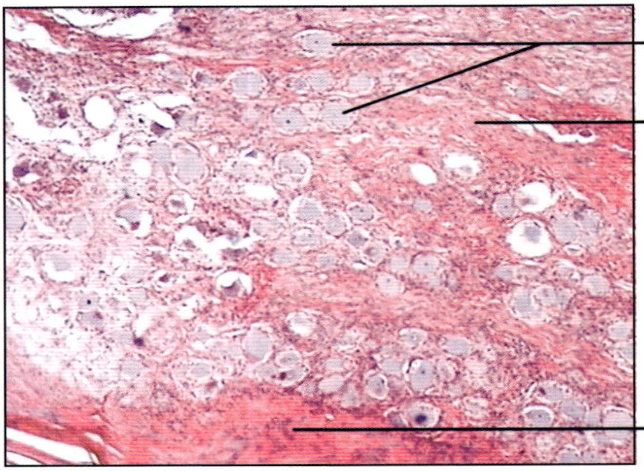

FIGURE 6.4 Dorsal root ganglion, H & E, X40

In the section under high power (Fig. 6.6), the cytoplasm and the round nuclei with the nucleoli of the unipolar neurons are visible. Each cell body is surrounded by two layers of cell capsules. The inner cell layer has smaller and flat epithelial cells, like satellite cells, present within the perineuronal space and closely surround the unipolar neurons. These cells continue with the Schwann cells, surrounding the axons. The outer cell layer forms the capsule cells of the connective tissue. Between the unipolar cells are the randomly arranged fibrocytes in connective tissue, which continue with the endoneurium of axons.

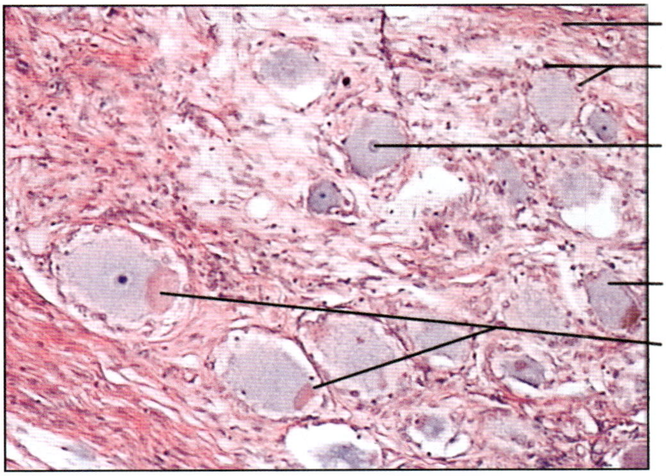

FIGURE 6.5 Dorsal root ganglion, H & E, X100

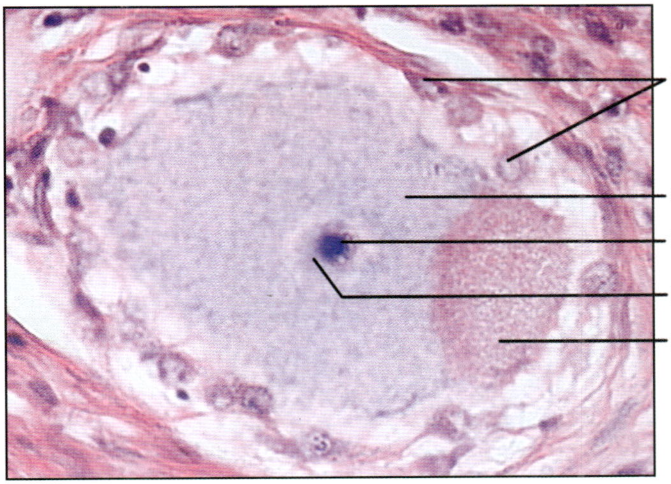

FIGURE 6.6 Dorsal root ganglion, H & E, X400

SYMPATHETIC GANGLION OR AUTONOMIC GANGLION

The neurons are multipolar, smaller and more uniform in size. The cells appear irregular because of the dendritic processes. Some cells do not show the nuclei since the section has not gone through the center. In aged individuals, lipofuscin pigment accumulates in the cytoplasm.

Section under scanner (Fig. 6.7) shows numerous multipolar cell bodies of the postganglionic sympathetic neurons. Discrete bundles of nerve fibers are randomly arranged.

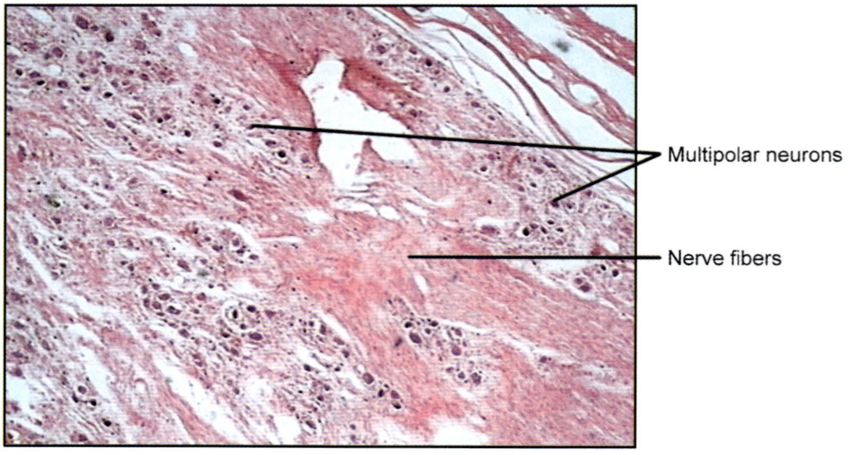

FIGURE 6.7 Sympathetic ganglion, H & E, X40

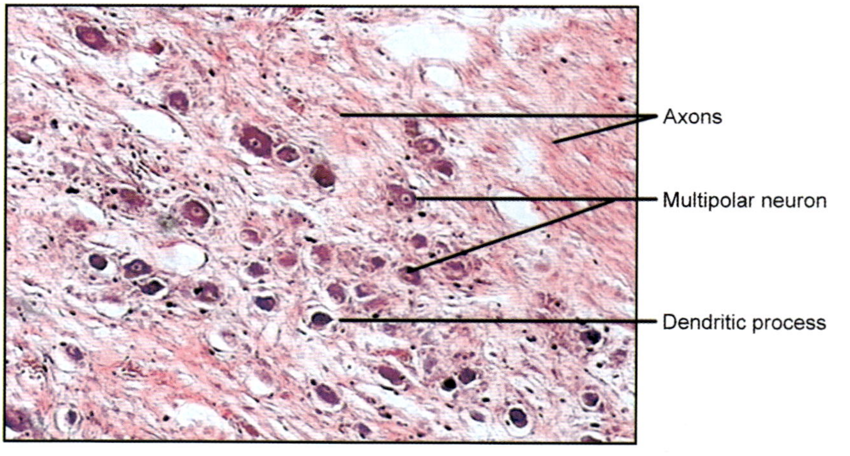

FIGURE 6.8 Sympathetic ganglion, H & E, X100

The section of low power (Fig. 6.8) shows the nuclei and the nucleoli in the cell bodies of the ganglion neurons. The processes of the cell bodies and the satellite cells are not clear in this section.

The section of high power (Fig. 6.9) shows clear nucleus and nucleolus, in the ganglion neurons. The satellite cells surrounding the cell bodies are less numerous compared to that of the spinal ganglion. The capsule cells are not well-defined. The satellite cells provide the structural and metabolic support to the neurons and insulate the neurons. The nerve axons aggregate into bundles and pass through the ganglion. The processes of the cell bodies are seen.

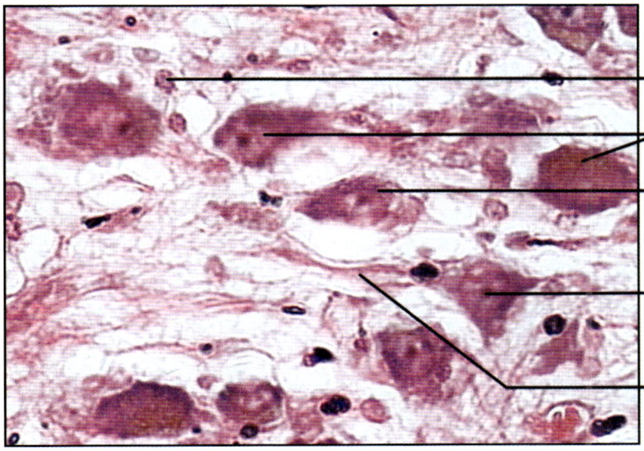

FIGURE 6.9 Sympathetic ganglion, H & E, X400

POINTS TO REMEMBER

Peripheral Nerve (TS)

- Nerve fibers are covered by epineurium, the fibrous dense connective tissue with blood vessels.
- Bundles of nerve fibers or fascicles are surrounded by perineurium, the connective tissue covering with a number of fibroblasts.
- Axon of each nerve fiber ensheathed by Schwann cell and endoneurium, the loose connective tissue with reticular fibers and fibroblasts.
- Diameter of the fibers is not uniform; some are fine, some are large and some with intermediate thickness.

Ganglia

Spinal/sensory/dorsal root and autonomic/sympathetic ganglia.

Type	*Spinal ganglia*	*Sympathetic ganglia*
Capsule	Thick	Thin
Neurons	Peripherally arranged, large and round pseudounipolar neurons	Irregularly arranged multipolar neurons appear star-shaped and are of varying sizes in sections
Nerve fibers	• Bundles of nerve fibers separate the neurons • Regularly arranged fibers enter and leave the ganglion	• Axons and dendrites pass through the widely-spaced neurons, without being involved in synapses • Irregularly scattered nerve fibers
Satellite cells	A layer of small cuboidal cells envelopes the neurons	Few satellite cells incompletely surround the cell body
Example	Dorsal root ganglia of the spinal nerves, sensory ganglia of cranial nerves (V, VII, IX, X)	• Sympathetic ganglia along sympathetic chain, • Otic/ciliary/submandibular/pterygopalatine ganglia

CHAPTER

7

Vascular Tissue

The vascular system consists of heart, major arteries, arterioles, capillaries, venules and veins. The main function is to deliver oxygenated blood to cells and tissues and to return venous blood to the lungs for gaseous exchange.

ARTERIES

Three types of arteries are the elastic arteries, muscular arteries and arterioles. Elastic arteries are the largest blood vessels in the body, the pulmonary trunk and aorta with its major branches (brachiocephalic, common carotid, subclavian and common iliac arteries). During blood flow, the elastic fibers present in large amount in the wall provide great resilience and flexibility. Muscular arteries, numerous in the body have the smooth muscle fibers in large number in their wall form the distributing arteries of the body. Arterioles are the smallest branches and the walls consist of one to five layers of smooth muscle fibers. Arterioles pass blood to the capillaries, the 'microscopic' blood vessels connecting arterioles and smallest veins or the venules.

VEINS

Venules usually accompany the arterioles and are formed by the union of the capillaries. The blood flows to postcapillary venules and then into small, medium and large (superior and inferior vena cavae) veins. Veins have typically thinner walls, larger diameters of the lumen and greater structural variation, when compared to the arteries. The small and medium sized veins present in the extremities have valves, which prevent the reflux of the blood. Valves are absent in the veins of central nervous system (CNS), superior and inferior vena cavae and in viscera.

GENERAL ARRANGEMENT OF THE LAYERS IN THE WALLS OF THE ARTERIES AND VEINS

From the lumen towards outside, the layers are the tunica intima, tunica media and tunica adventitia.

Tunica intima is the innermost layer consisting of single layer of squamous epithelium, the endothelium; surrounding it is the basal lamina of the endothelial cells and subendothelial layer with loose connective tissue and occasional smooth muscle cells. In arteries, subendothelial layer contains fenestrated lamella of elastic material, called the internal elastic membrane.

Tunica media is the middle layer consisting of smooth muscle cells arranged in circumferential manner. It is relatively thick in arteries when compared to the veins. The other constituents of tunica media are elastin, reticular fibers. The external elastic membrane separates the tunica media from the tunica adventitia.

Tunica adventitia is the outermost layer composed of longitudinally arranged collagen tissue and few elastic fibers, which gradually merge with the loose connective tissue, surrounding the vessel. Tunica adventitia is quite thin in arteries and thick in veins. Small vessels present in this layer in large arteries and veins are called vasa vasorum, which supply blood to the outer part of the walls and a network of autonomic nerves, the nervi vascularis control the contraction of smooth muscle cells.

MUSCULAR ARTERY OR MEDIUM-SIZED ARTERY

The tunica media is thick and contains more smooth muscle fibers and less elastic fibers. The characteristic features of these arteries are the internal elastic membrane, which separates the tunica intima from the tunica media and external elastic membrane, which separates the tunica media from the tunica adventitia. Most of the arteries in the body belong to the muscular artery. The tunica media is thick in the artery when compared to the accompanying vein.

In the section under scanner (Fig. 7.1), the internal elastic lamina is identified, separating the tunica intima and tunica media. The tunica media is almost same as the thickness of tunica adventitia.

In the section under low power (Fig. 7.2), the nuclei of the endothelium are not appreciated. The internal elastic lamina between the tunica intima and tunica media is seen. In tunica media, abundant smooth muscle cells are visible. The cut sections of the longitudinally running collagen fibers in tunica adventitia are seen. External elastic lamina is present on the periphery of the tunica media.

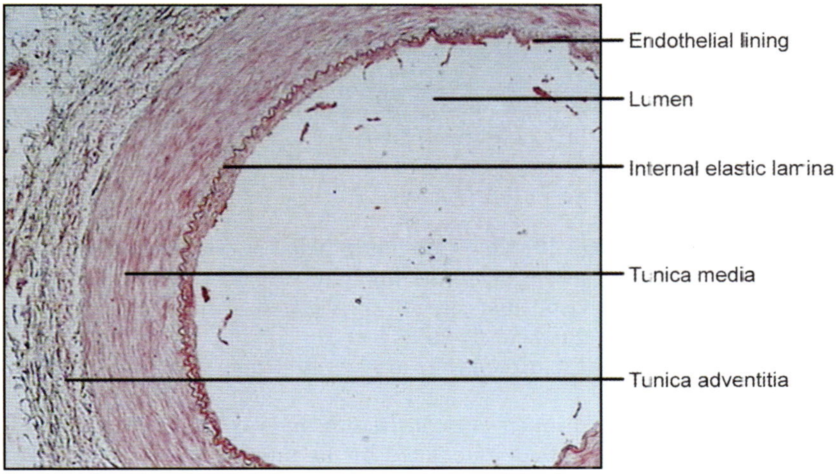

FIGURE 7.1 Muscular artery, H & E, X40

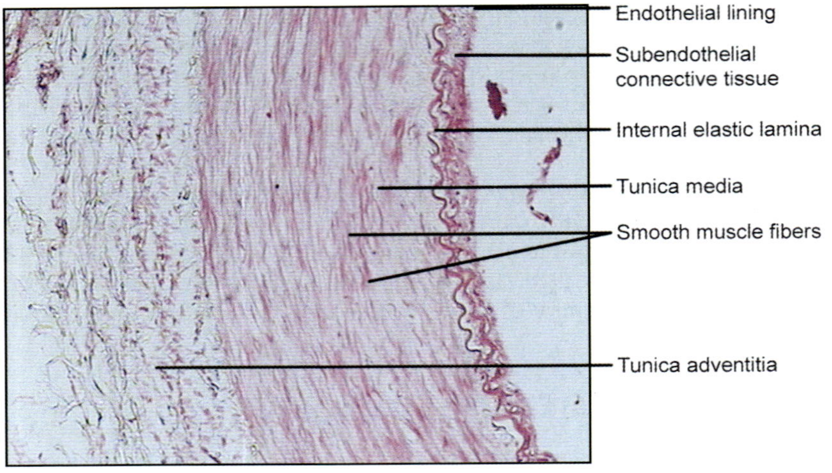

FIGURE 7.2 Muscular artery, H & E, X100

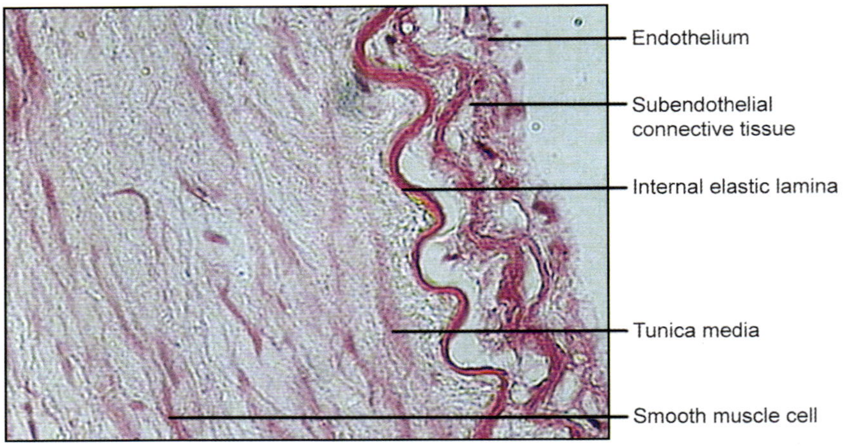

FIGURE 7.3 Muscular artery, H & E, X400

Section under high power (Fig. 7.3) shows the endothelial and subendothelial layers of the tunica intima. The tunica media of several layers of smooth muscle fibers arranged in circular layers is visible. The thin dark strands of elastic fibers are not appreciated. Tunica adventitia contains light stained collagen fibers and dark stained elastic fibers.

In the accompanying vein, all the three layers are less in proportion, when compared to the artery.

Blood flow and blood pressure through vasoconstriction and vasodilation are controlled by the high proportion of smooth muscle fibers innervated by the unmyelinated axons of sympathetic system.

LARGE ARTERY OR ELASTIC ARTERY

Elastic arteries are known as conducting arteries. In large artery, the bulk of tunica media is formed by elastic fibers; smooth muscle fibers are less abundant. The elastic fibers resist the pressure variations and allow the steady flow of blood in the respective arteries. In elastic arteries, the tunica media occupies most of the walls of the vessel; whereas the tunica adventitia is reduced to a small area. In the tunica adventitia, venules of different sizes and arterioles are present, to supply the connective tissue and are known as vasa vasorum.

The elastic arteries transport blood from the heart and along the systemic vascular path. During systole, when a large volume of blood is ejected from the ventricles into the lumen, the increased number of elastic fibers in the walls allows the elastic arteries to greatly expand in diameter. During diastole, the expanded elastic walls recoil on the blood in the lumen and force it to move forward through the vascular channels. As a result, a less variable systemic blood pressure is maintained and blood flows more evenly through the body, during heartbeats.

In this section under scanner (Fig. 7.4), the three layers are identified. Tunica intima is identified by its endothelial layer. Tunica media is the large layer, extending through the thickness of the wall. Tunica adventitia is small and hardly visible. Few elastic fibers present in the adventitia, but it consists of longitudinally running collagen fibers.

In the section of low power (Fig. 7.5), the endothelial and subendothelial layers are quite distinct. The tunica media has smooth muscle cells with large amount of elastic fibers, which are not distinctly seen in H and E preparation. In special stained preparations, like resorcin-fuchsin, the elastic lamellae appear to be interrupted, which are actually the fenestrations or openings.

Section under high power (Fig. 7.6) shows the nuclei of the endothelial cells and subendothelial cells of the tunica intima. The nuclei seen in the tunica media are of smooth muscle fibers wound spirally between the elastic membranes.

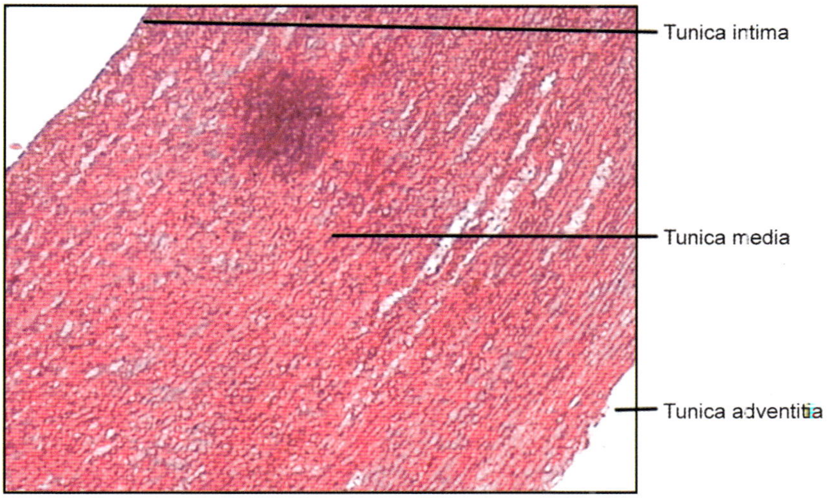

FIGURE 7.4 Large artery, H & E, X40

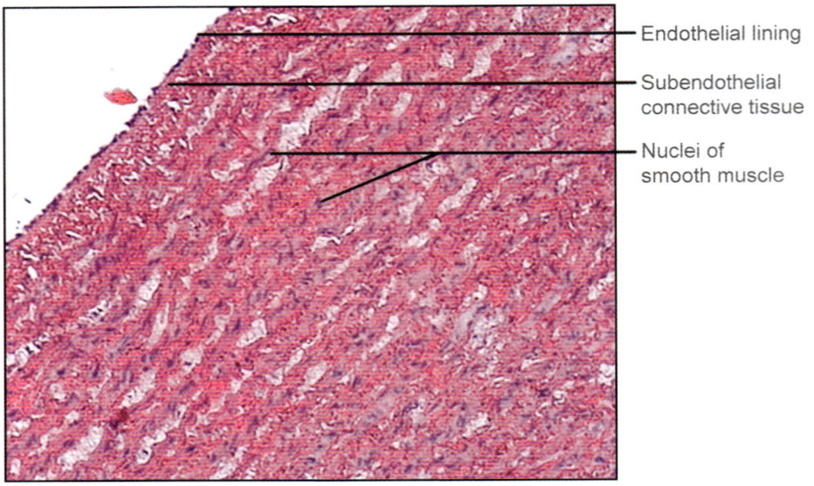

FIGURE 7.5 Large artery, H & E, X100

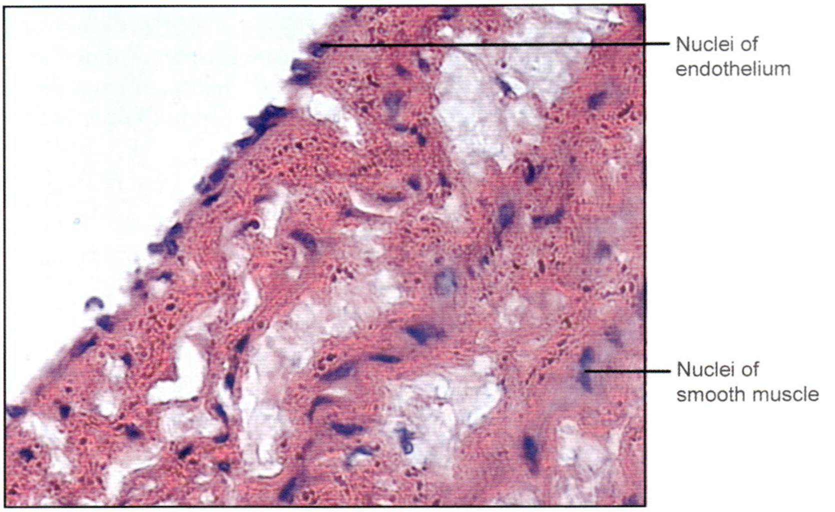

FIGURE 7.6 Large artery, H & E, X400

LARGE VEIN

The wall of large vein has a thick muscular tunica adventitia with longitudinally oriented smooth muscle fibers. In TS the muscle fibers are seen as segregated bundles. Vasa vasorum are present in tunica adventitia. The tunica media is thinner and compact when compared to the adventitia.

In veins, the blood pressure is lower than in arteries. Venous blood flow is passive. In the head and trunk, venous blood flow primarily results from negative pressure in the thoracic and abdominal cavities and also because of the respiratory movements. Venous blood return from the extremities is

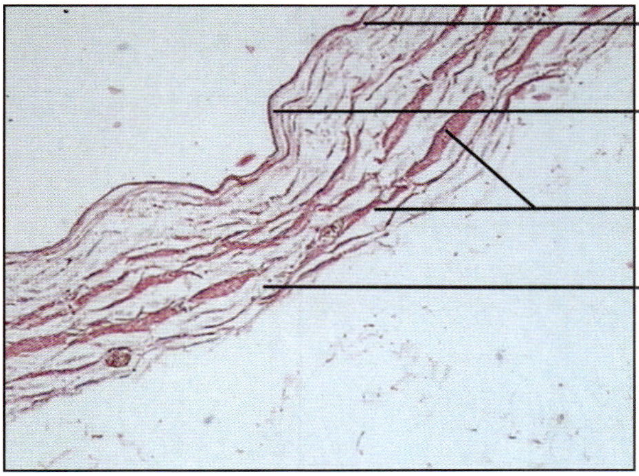

FIGURE 7.7 Large vein, H & E, X40

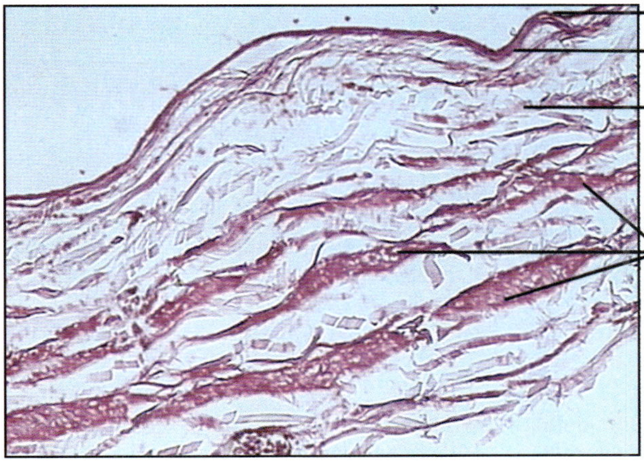

FIGURE 7.8 Large vein, H & E, X100

aided by the contraction of muscles surrounding the veins and the venous valves present in relation to the tunica intima and the lumen.

The three layers of the wall are distinguished in the section shown under scanner (Fig. 7.7) . The boundary between the tunica intima and the tunica media not distinctly separated. Subendothelial connective tissue is thin.

Section under low power (Fig. 7.8), the nuclei of the endothelium are not appreciated. The tunica media is thin consisting of smooth muscle cells, collagen fibers and few fibroblasts arranged circumferentially. The tunica adventitia, the thickest of the layers in the large vein has collagen and elastic fibers, fibroblasts and longitudinally running smooth muscle cells.

In the section under high power (Fig. 7.9), the nuclei of the endothelium are well-appreciated. The smooth muscle cells in tunica media are arranged circumferentially. The tunica adventitia is very thick.

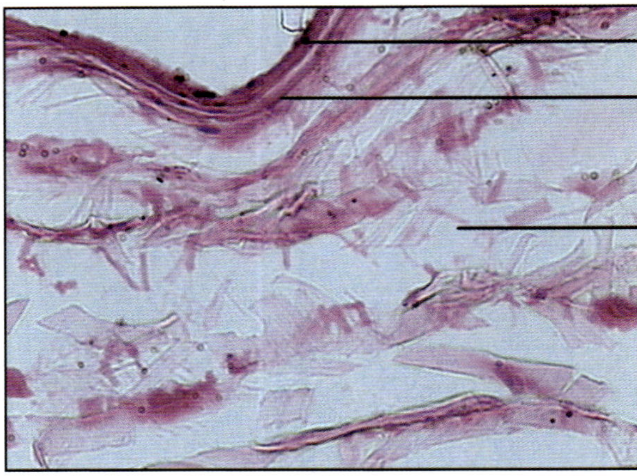

FIGURE 7.9 Large vein, H & E, X400

POINTS TO REMEMBER

Types	*Medium-sized artery*	*Large artery*	*Large vein*
Tunica intima: • Endothelium	Endothelial cells with basal lamina	Thick lining endothelium with basal lamina	Endothelial layer with basal lamina
• Subendothelial CT	Sparse	• Well-defined with collagen and elastic fibers and smooth muscle cells • Fibroblasts absent	Thin, but also with smooth muscle cells
• Internal elastic membrane (fenestrated membrane of Henle)	Well-defined wavy structure	Present, but not distinct	Not distinct
Tunica media	• Mainly of smooth muscle cells with intervening collagen, reticular and elastic fibers • Few or no fibroblasts	• Thickest of the 3 layers • Abundant elastic fibers with intervening smooth muscle cells, collagen fibers and ground substance • Elastic fibers in the form of membranes	Thin consisting of smooth muscle cells, collagen fibers and fibroblasts
Tunica adventitia	• As thick as tunica media • Mainly collagen fibers • Adjacent to tunica media form prominent external elastic lamina	• Less than half the thickness of tunica media • Mainly of collagen fibers with loose network of elastic fibers • Fibroblasts and macrophages present • Vasa vasorum seen	• Thickest consisting of longitudinally running smooth muscle cells • Fibroblasts, collagen and elastic fibers seen • Vasa vasorum extends up to the tunica media
Lumen	Round and intact	Round and intact	• Collapsed and irregular • Larger lumen than the artery
Example	Radial, ulnar, tibial	Aorta, pulmonary trunk	Superior vena cava, inferior vena cava, portal vein

CHAPTER

8

Lymphatic Tissue

The function of lymphoid system is to collect excess interstitial fluid into lymphatic capillaries, transport absorbed lipids from the small intestine and respond immunologically to invading foreign substances.

The lymphatic system consists of groups of cells, tissues and organs that monitor body surfaces and internal fluid compartments to react to the presence of potentially harmful substances. Lymphocytes are the definitive cell type of the lymphatic system and are the effector cells in the response of the immune system to the harmful substances.

Lymphatic system includes the diffuse lymphatic tissue, lymphatic nodules, lymph nodes, spleen, bone marrow, thymus, mucosa-associated lymphatic tissue (MALT) (tonsils) and gut-associated lymphatic tissue (GALT) (solitary lymphatic follicles in jejunum, Peyer's patch in ileum, vermiform appendix). The various lymphatic organs and lymphatic tissues are often collectively referred to as the immune system. Lymphatic system is also considered as part of the vascular system. Lymphatic tissues serve as sites where lymphocytes proliferate, differentiate and mature. Lymphocytes are sensitized to recognize and destroy specific antigens. The immunocompetent cells distinguish between self (molecules normally present within an organism) and nonself (foreign molecules, those not normally present) molecules.

LYMPH NODE

Lymph nodes are small, encapsulated lymphatic organs located in the path of the lymph vessels. Lymph nodes consist of dense masses of lymphocyte aggregations, intermixed with dilated lymphatic sinuses containing lymph and supported by a framework of fine reticular fibers. The main function is phagocytosis. Lymph nodes filter the lymph and acts as the principal site in which T- and B-lymphocytes undergo antigen-dependent proliferation and differentiation into effector lymphocytes (plasma cells and T-cells) and memory B-cells.

Lymph nodes produce, store and recirculate B- and T-lymphocytes. The B-lymphocytes are present in the lymphatic nodules, whereas T-lymphocytes are present below the nodules and in the deep or paracortical region. Lymph node is divided into outer cortex and inner medulla. The connective tissue capsule surrounds the lymph node and sends trabeculae into the cortex. Cortex consists of lymphatic nodules, lymphatic sinuses and lymph channels. Medulla consists of medullary cords and medullary sinuses. There are three sinuses in lymph node—subcapsular

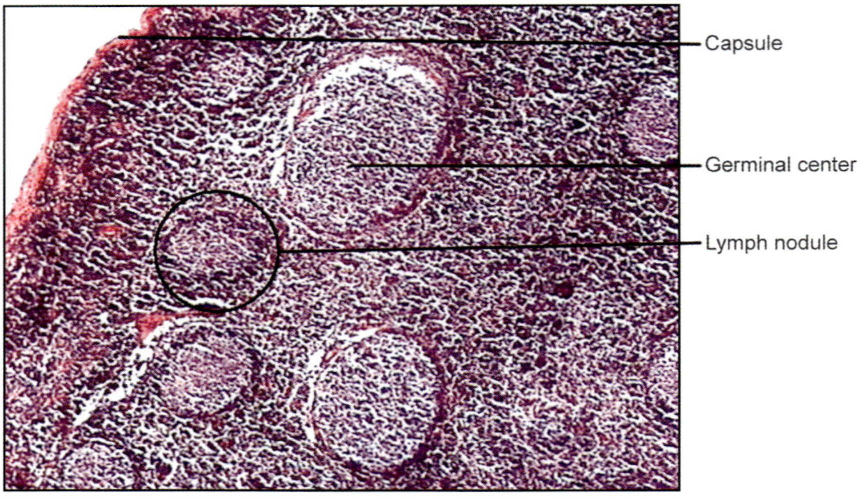

FIGURE 8.1 Lymph node, H & E, X40

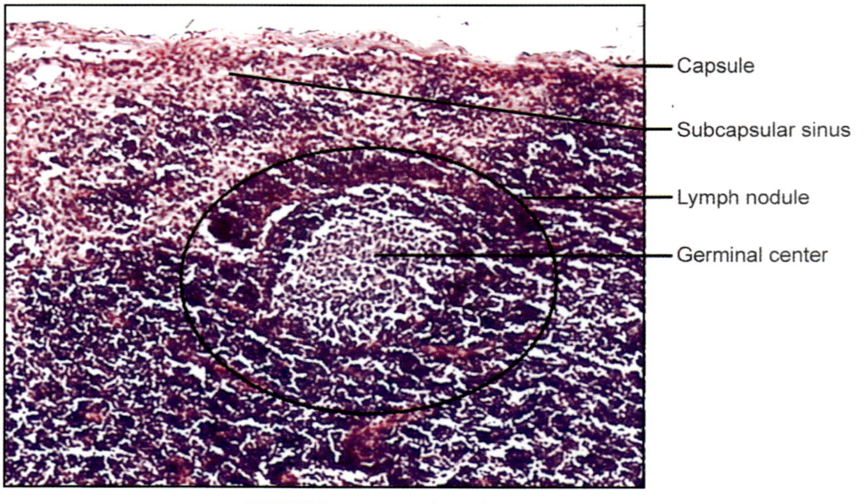

FIGURE 8.2 Lymph node, H & E, X100

sinus just beneath the capsule, trabecular sinus around the trabeculae and medullary sinus in medulla. The lymph flow is from afferent lymphatic vessels→subcapsular sinus→trabecular sinus→medullary sinus→efferent lymphatic vessels in hilum.

Section under scanner (Fig. 8.1) shows the cortex of the lymph node. The capsule is composed of dense connective tissue from which trabeculae penetrate into the organ. The cortex contains the lymphatic nodules and a deeper part without nodules is the paracortex or deep cortex.

The medulla (not seen in the picture) is characterized by narrow strands of anastomozing lymphatic tissue containing numerous lymphocytes and the medullary cords separated by light appearing areas known as the medullary sinuses.

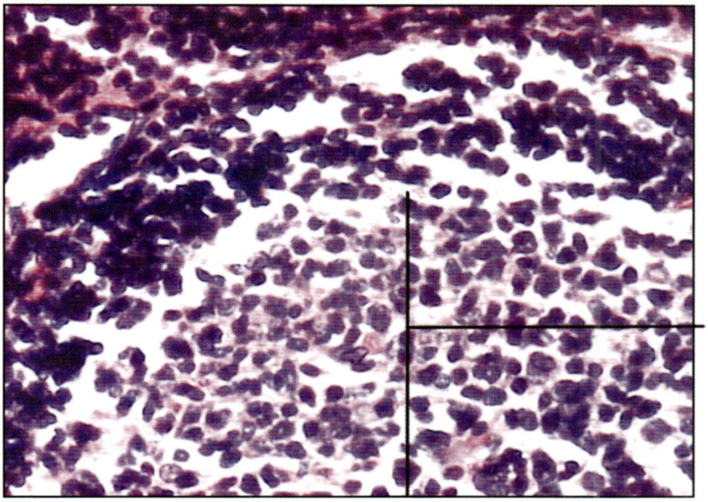

FIGURE 8.3 Lymph node, H & E, X400

Section under low power (Fig. 8.2) shows the cortical or subcapsular sinus and trabecular sinuses immediately below the capsule and trabeculae. The sinus receive lymph from the afferent lymphatic vessels; which penetrate the capsule.

Section under high power (Fig. 8.3) of the lymphatic nodule is sectioned through the center. As seen in the picture, the center of the lymphatic nodule is light stained and is known as the germinal center containing large and medium-sized lymphocytes. The germinal center is the active site of lymphocyte proliferation.

THYMUS

Thymus is a lobulated lymphatic organ enclosed by the connective tissue capsule. The histology of thymus shows age changes. Thymus attains its greatest development just after birth. Thymus starts by puberty a gradual regression and degeneration; the lymphocyte production declines and the thymic corpuscles become more prominent. The parenchyma (cellular portion) is replaced by loose connective tissue and fat (adipose) cells.

Section under scanner (Fig. 8.4) exhibits adipose tissue accumulation and signs of involution associated with the increase in age.

Thymus is surrounded by a connective tissue capsule, which sends trabeculae into the parenchyma to form the thymic lobules. The lobules are incomplete because of the discontinuous nature of the trabeculae. The lobules are seen dividing into dark stained cortex and light stained medulla. The trabeculae are incomplete; hence, medulla is continuous with the adjacent lobules. The cortex contains numerous densely packed lymphocytes, whereas medulla has less densely packed lymphocytes, more epithelial reticular cells and numerous thymic (Hassall's) corpuscles. Thymic corpuscles are the characteristic feature of thymus. The lymphocytes and epithelial reticular cells form the bulk of the organ.

Sections under low (Fig. 8.5) and high power (Fig. 8.6) show that the thymic corpuscles are oval structures consisting of round aggregations of flattened epithelial cells. The center of the corpuscles stained pink, since the epithelial cells calcify or degenerate. Thymic corpuscles secrete cytokines.

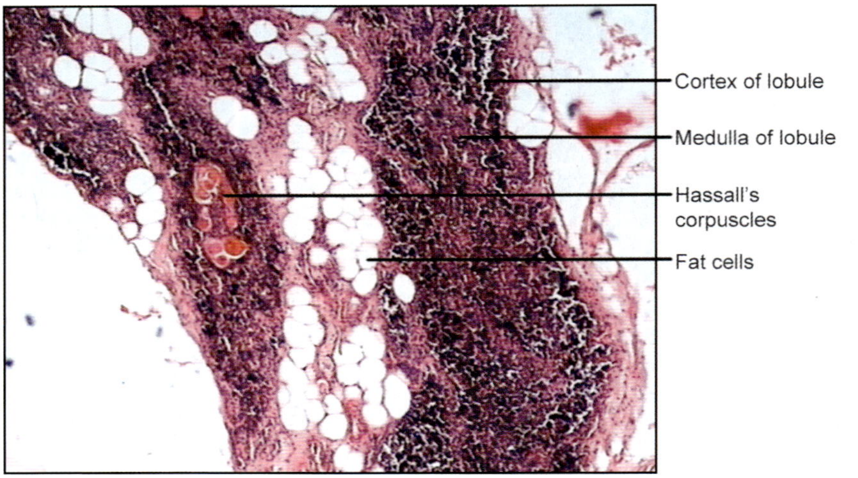

FIGURE 8.4 Thymus, H & E, X40

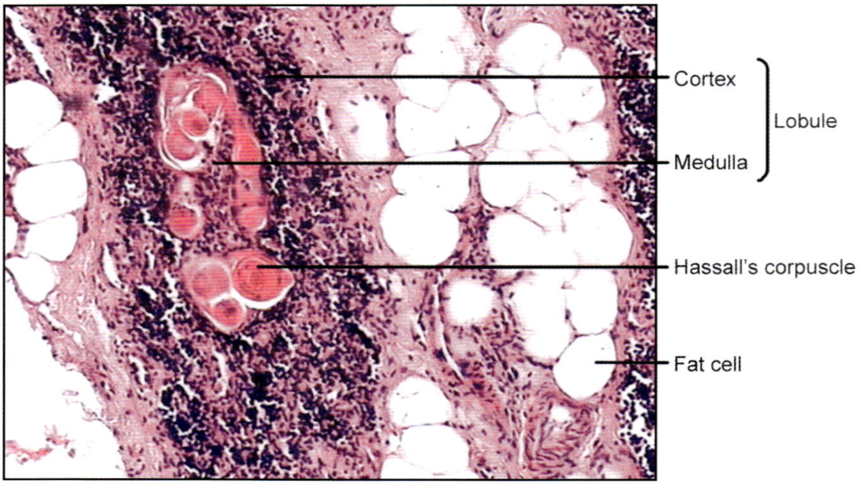

FIGURE 8.5 Thymus, H & E, X100

TONSIL

Palatine tonsils, the paired, ovoid structures consist of dense accumulations of lymphatic tissue located in mucous membrane, at the junction of oropharynx and oral cavity. Palatine tonsils guard the opening of the pharynx, the common entry to respiratory and digestive tracts.

Section under scanner (Figs 8.7A and B) shows the general features of the palatine tonsil. Tonsil has an attached and a free surface. The picture shows the free surface covered by the stratified squamous nonkeratinized epithelium. In numerous places, the epithelium dips into the

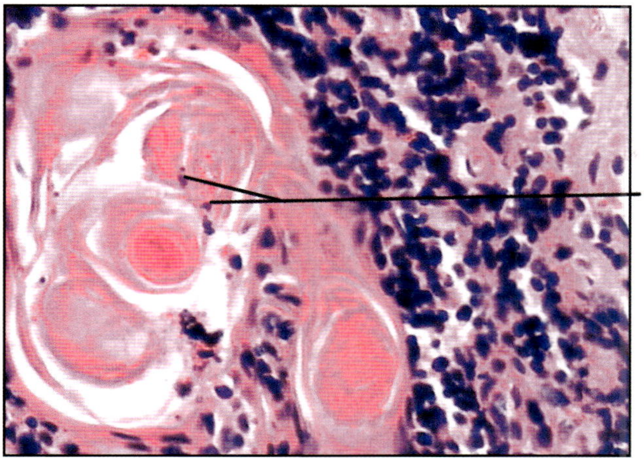

FIGURE 8.6 Thymus, H & E, X400

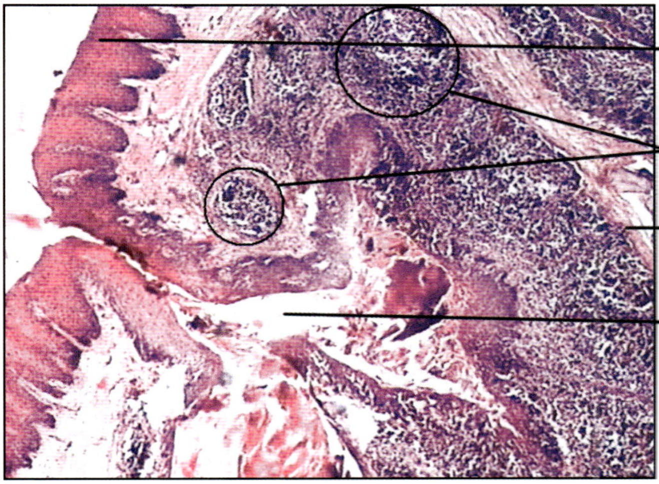

FIGURE 8.7A Tonsil: Free surface, H & E, X40

underlying connective tissue forming tonsillar crypts, which are also lined by stratified squamous nonkeratinized epithelium. The lumen of crypt contains desquamated epithelial cells and bacteria. Surrounding the tonsillar crypts are present the lymphatic nodules and diffuse lymphatic tissue in the connective tissue.

The attached surface of the palatine tonsil has a dense connective tissue forming the capsule. The connective tissue trabeculae arise from the capsule and pass towards the free surface between the lymphatic nodules. The capsule usually acts as barrier against spreading tonsillar infections. Beneath the capsule are the mucous glands and skeletal muscle fibers.

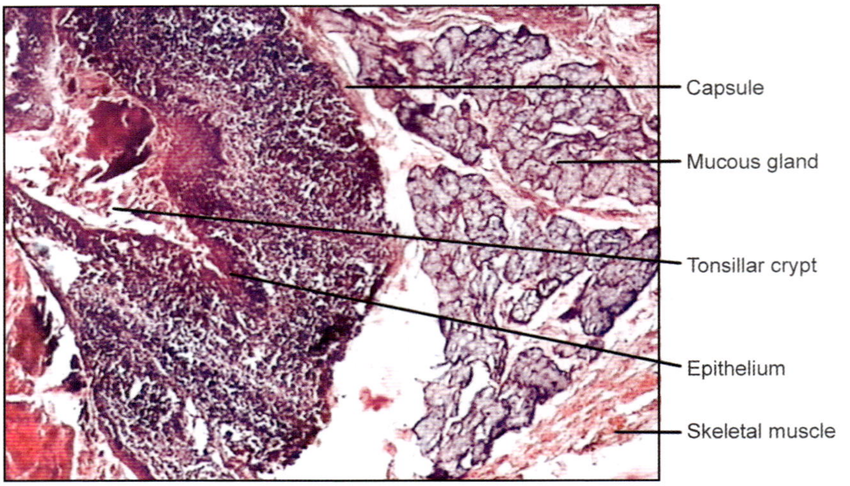

FIGURE 8.7B Tonsil: Attached surface, H & E, X40

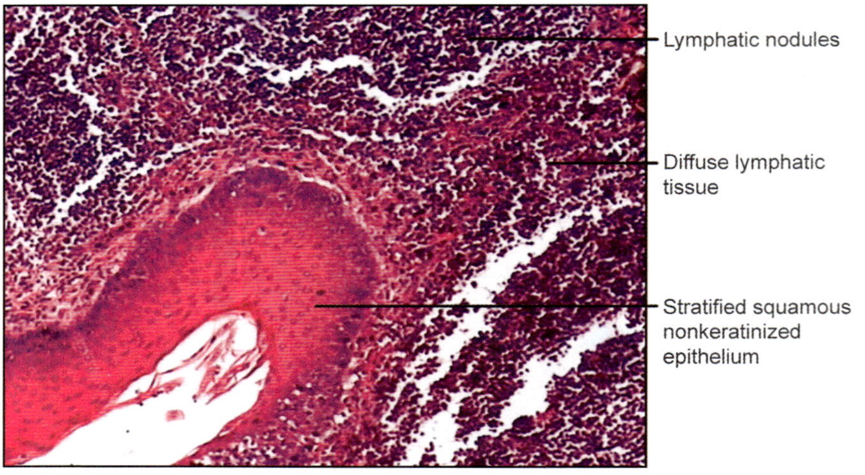

FIGURE 8.8 Tonsil, H & E, X100

Sections under low power (Fig. 8.8) and high power (Figs 8.9A and B) show the different layers of stratified squamous non-keratinized epithelium, diffuse (free) lymphatic tissue and lymphatic nodules. The epithelium may be often infiltrated with lymphocytes and therefore, it may be difficult to recognize the epithelium.

SPLEEN

Spleen is the largest lymphatic organ with an extensive blood supply. Spleen is surrounded by a capsule. Spleen filters blood and is the site of immune responses to blood-borne antigens. Spleen

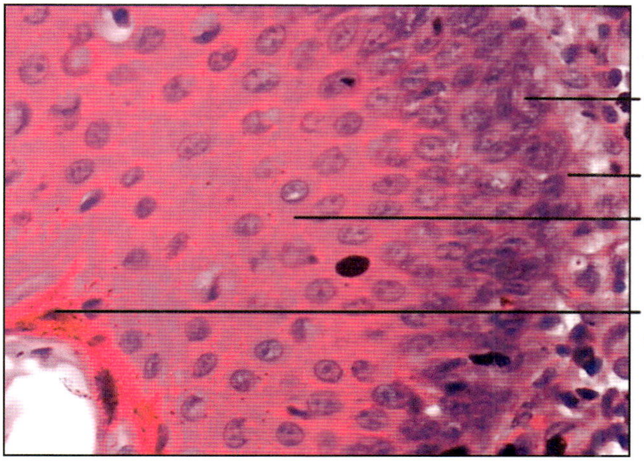

FIGURE 8.9A Tonsil, H & E X400

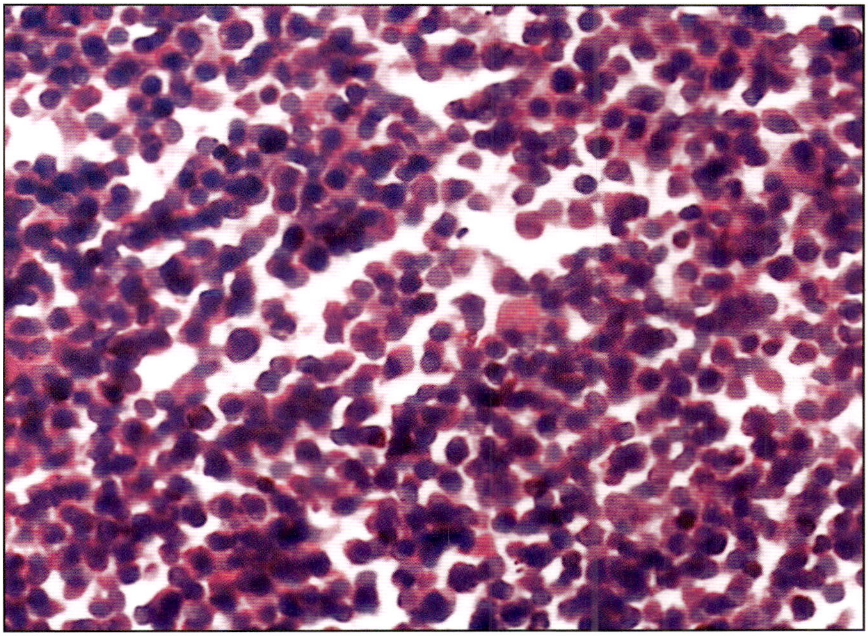

FIGURE 8.9B Tonsil, H & E X400

does not show the distinct cortex and medulla. Spleen consists of red pulp and white pulp, so named because of the appearance, in the preparation of the fresh tissue.

Section under scanner (Fig. 8.10) shows the dense irregular connective tissue capsule and the two major components of spleen, red pulp and white pulp along with the cut sections of trabeculae.

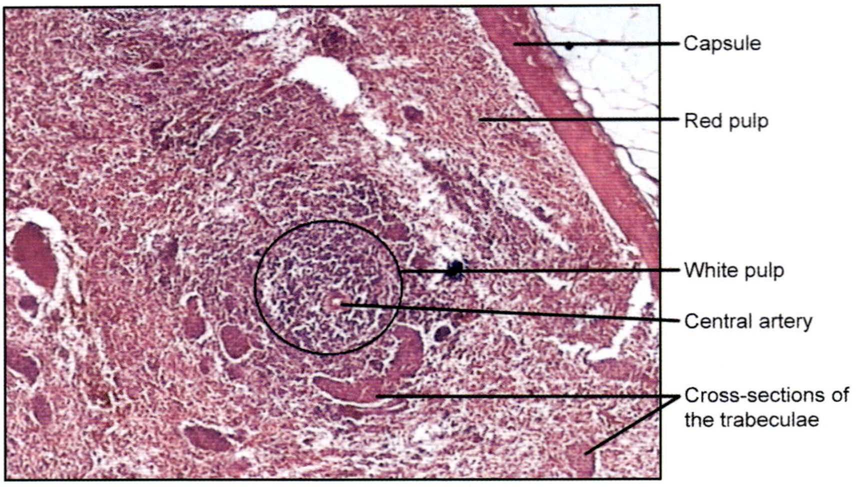

FIGURE 8.10 Spleen, H & E, X40

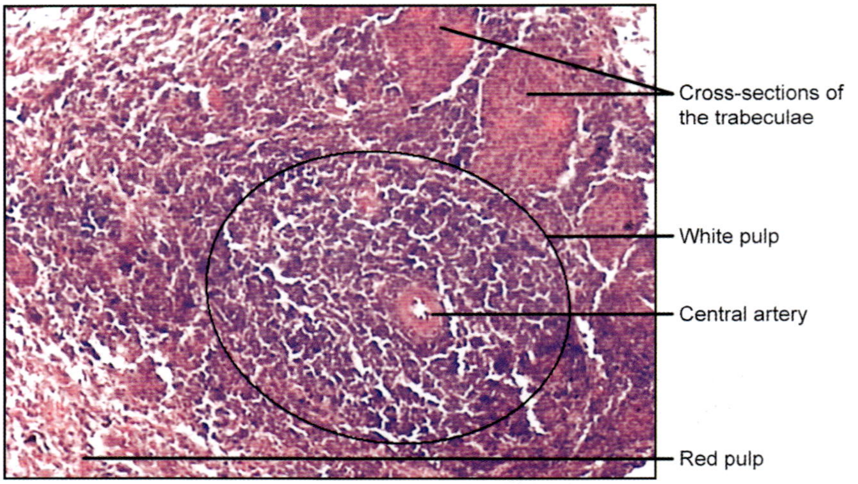

FIGURE 8.11 Spleen, H & E, X100

The red pulp forms the greater bulk of the splenic tissue. The name red pulp is given, since it is red 'in life' as a result of natural coloration of the numerous red blood cells. The white pulp gets the name because the lymphocytes appear white 'in life'. The lymphocytes ensheathe the blood vessel, the central artery. The lymphatic tissue surrounding the artery undergoes periodic expansion forming the nodules and during the process, the central artery is displaced peripherally within the nodule.

Section under low power (Fig. 8.11) shows two elements in the red pulp, venous sinuses and splenic cords of Billroth between the sinuses. Venous sinuses are dilated vessels lined with modified endothelium of elongated cells. Splenic cords are aggregations of reticular fibers, small lymphocytes,

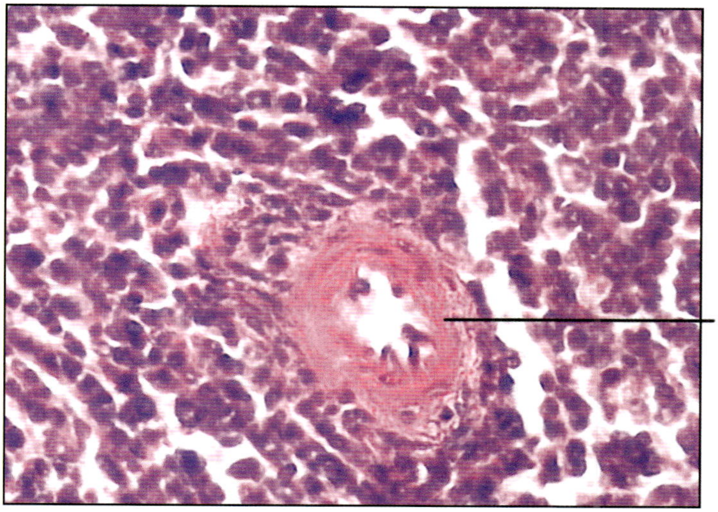

FIGURE 8.12 Spleen, H & E, X400

erythrocytes, plasma cells, macrophages and other granulocytes. Pulp arteries, capillaries and pulp veins also form part of red pulp. The main function of red pulp is to filter antigens, microorganisms, platelets and aged or abnormal erythrocytes from the blood.

In the section, it is seen, that the lymphatic tissue is not in the nodular form; present as a cuff around the central artery called the periarteriolar lymphatic sheath.

Section under high power (Fig. 8.12) shows, white pulp along with the central artery. White pulp mainly consists of lymphatic tissue. Lymphatic cells that surround the central artery are T-lymphocytes, whereas the lymphatic nodules contain mainly B-lymphocytes. Antigen presenting cells and macrophages are also present within the white pulp; cells detect trapped bacteria and antigens and initiate immune response against the bacteria. T-lymphocytes and B-lymphocytes interact, activate, proliferate and perform immune responses.

POINTS TO REMEMBER

Lymph Node

- Located in the course of the afferent and efferent lymphatic vessels.
- The only lymphatic organ containing lymph sinuses.
- Usually oval or bean-shaped and has hilum.
- Covered by capsule (collagen and elastic fibers). Trabeculae extend into the substance of the organ.
- Lymph node divides into outer cortex and inner medulla.
- *Cortex*: Primary lymphatic nodules, secondary follicles with pale stained germinal centers and subcapsular and peritrabecular sinuses. Sinus spaces lined by reticuloendothelial cells and traversed by reticular cells and fibers.
- *Medulla*: Irregularly arranged medullary cords and sinuses.

- Lymph flows from afferent lymph vessels to the subcapsular → peritrabecular → medullary sinuses and through hilum to the efferent lymph vessels.
- *Cells*: B-lymphocytes [lymphatic nodules; antibody production (humoral immunity)], T-lymphocytes [in between nodules and medullary cords; cytotoxic (cell-mediated immunity)], macrophages (lymph sinuses, around walls of lymph sinuses and germinal centers, numerous in medulla than cortex; antigen presenting cells).

Thymus

- Primary or central lymphoid organ.
- Distinct but incompletely separated lobules formed by trabeculae, derived from the connective tissue capsule.
- Each lobule divided into a peripheral dense zone, the cortex and a light stained central zone, the medulla, which is continuous with the adjacent lobules.
- In lobules, central part homogeneous, peripheral part concentrically arranged cells.
- *Cortex*: Mainly small lymphocytes.
- *Medulla*: Young lymphocytes, lymphoblasts, reticuloepithelial cells and pink stained rounded masses, Hassall's corpuscles. Hassall's corpuscles are concentrically arranged flattened or polygonal reticuloepithelial cells present around the completely degenerated hyaline mass.
- *Cells*: T-lymphocytes/Thymocytes (cortex, medulla; T-helper cells/cytotoxic T-cells), epithelial cells (internal surface of capsule, surface of septa and blood vessels; thymic hormone), macrophages (associated to capsule, corticomedullary junction, medulla; phagocytic).

Tonsil

- Attached and free surfaces.
- Attached surface has the capsule of connective tissue, thereby tonsil is adhered to the surrounding structures. Mucous glands present in the submucosa or in the connective tissue next to the capsule.
- Free surface lined by the nonkeratinized stratified squamous epithelium. At various places deep indentations or pockets occur as tonsillar crypts lined by the surface epithelium.
- Lymphatic nodules in the lamina propria, surround each crypt.
- Example for mucosa associated lymphoid tissue (MALT).

Spleen

- Encapsulated in a dense irregular connective tissue capsule, which is covered by the mesothelium. From the capsule trabeculae extend into the parenchyma of the spleen (splenic pulp).
- Splenic pulp, 2 different regions:
  - *White pulp*: Lymphatic nodules and periarteriolar lymphatic tissue (T- and B-cells).
  - *Red pulp*: Plexus of venous sinuses (splenic sinuses) separated by anastomozing cords (pulp cords, cords of Billroth) consisting of diffuse lymphocytes, erythrocytes, endothelial cells, stave cells, T-cells, B-cells and macrophages (giant cells of spleen).

CHAPTER

9

Glandular Tissue

There are three major salivary glands: Parotid, submandibular and sublingual. The glands are located outside the oral cavity and convey their secretions into the mouth through large excretory ducts. The glands are classified as compound tubuloacinar glands.

The glands are composed of cellular secretory units, the acini and numerous excretory ducts. The acini are small, sac-like dilations located at the end of the first part of the excretory duct system called the intercalated ducts. They are surrounded by the connective tissue, which gives septa to divide the gland into lobes and lobules.

Two types of cells are present in the salivary glands: Serous and mucous cells. Serous cells are pyramidal in shape. The spherical or round nuclei are present between the center and the basement membrane. The apical part is filled with secretory granules.

Mucous cells are similar to serous cells, but the cytoplasm is filled with light staining secretion called mucus. Because of the accumulation of the mucus, the nucleus is flattened and displaced towards the basement membrane.

In some glands, both mucous and serous cells are present in the same acinus where mucous cells predominate and serous cells form a crescent-or moon-shaped cap over the mucous cells. These crescent-shaped serous cells are the serous demilunes. The secretions from serous cells in the demilunes enter the lumen through tiny intercellular canaliculi between the mucous cells.

Some flattened cells surrounding both the serous and mucous acini and present between the cells and the basement membrane are the myoepithelial cells. These cells are highly branched and contractile and surround the acini like a basket and because of this nature, are also known as basket cells. Secretory products are expelled from the acini by the contraction of myoepithelial cells.

Serous, mucous and mixed glands empty the secretions initially into the intercalated ducts, which are smallest ducts lined by the low cuboidal epithelium. Myoepithelial cells surround some parts of the intercalated ducts. Several intercalated ducts merge to form larger striated ducts, lined by columnar epithelium exhibiting tiny basal striations. The striations are the basal infoldings of cell membrane containing the mitochondria and cellular interdigitations. These striated ducts join to form the larger intralobular ducts, which inturn join to form the interlobular and interlobar ducts. These ducts at the terminal part are lined by stratified low cuboidal or columnar epithelium.

The salivary glands secrete saliva, the source of calcium, phosphate and antibodies. The functions of saliva are moistening dry foods, dissolving and suspending food, buffering the oral contents, digestion of carbohydrates and controlling the bacterial flora.

Contents of saliva are water, proteins, glycoproteins (enzymes-lysosome and salivary/alpha amylase; antibodies) and electrolytes (potassium, sodium, calcium, phosphorus, chloride).

SEROUS SALIVARY GLAND

Parotid salivary gland is a large serous salivary gland. The gland is surrounded by connective tissue capsule from which arise numerous septa that subdivide the gland into lobes and lobules. In the septa are arterioles, venules, interlobular excretory ducts and adipose cells. Each lobule consists of serous acini. The cytoplasm is slightly basophilic and the lumen of some of the acini not always visible. At higher magnification small secretory granules (zymogen granules) are seen in cell apices.

The serous cells secrete poorly or nonglycosylated protein (antimicrobial, protective) which is watery in nature and salivary amylase (initiates hydrolyses of carbohydrates).

Section under scanner (Fig. 9.1) shows the lobules separated by the connective tissue septa. Each lobule shows serous acini and intralobular ducts. The intercalated ducts are difficult to be identified. Blood vessels are seen in the connective tissue septa.

Section under low power shows (Fig. 9.2) the connective tissue septa with blood vessels separating the lobules are observed. The excretory ducts (intralobular) are seen well.

From the section, under high power (Fig. 9.3) it is observed that the lumen of the acini is not regular. It is because, the lumen is smaller in size and also the variability of the section gone through the acini. The excretory duct is evident in the lower part of the section. The duct is lined by columnar epithelium and one part of the duct shows the striations.

MUCOUS SALIVARY GLAND

Sublingual gland is the mucous salivary gland. Both serous and mucous acini are present, but mucous acini predominate. The intercalated ducts are short or absent and are not observed in the section. The nonstriated interlobular excretory ducts are more prevalent. The intralobular excretory ducts are equivalent to the striated ducts of submandibular and parotid glands, but lack extensive membrane infolding and basal striations. Interlobular connective tissue septa are more abundant.

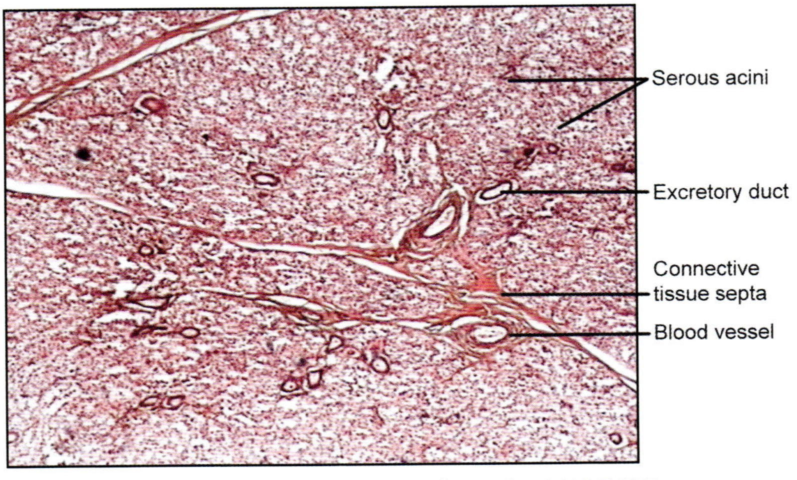

FIGURE 9.1 Serous salivary gland, H & E, X40

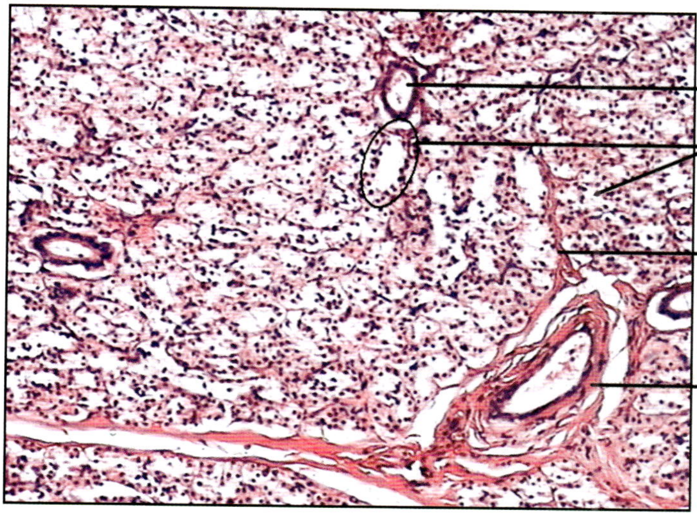

FIGURE 9.2 Serous salivary gland, H & E, X100

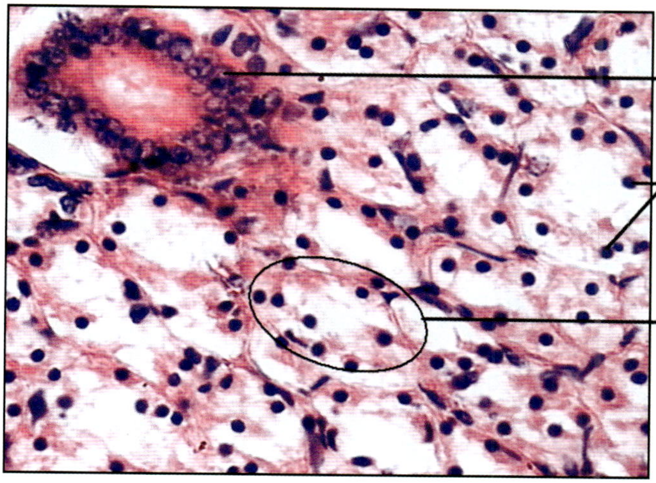

FIGURE 9.3 Serous salivary gland, H & E, X400

The mucous cells secrete viscous and slimy secretions.

The sections (Figs 9.4 and 9.5) show the structures under scanner and low power. The mucous acini are present in different sizes and shapes. The cells look frothy in appearance, since the secretory products are washed off during the preparation of the tissue. The nuclei are present in the base of the cells due to the accumulation of the secretion. Numerous excretory ducts are visible.

Section under high power (Fig. 9.6) shows the mucous acini clearly. The cells are empty and give frothy appearance, because the mucous secretion is lost during the tissue preparation. The round structures resembling water droplets are the air bubbles. The nuclei present at the base of the cells are clearly seen.

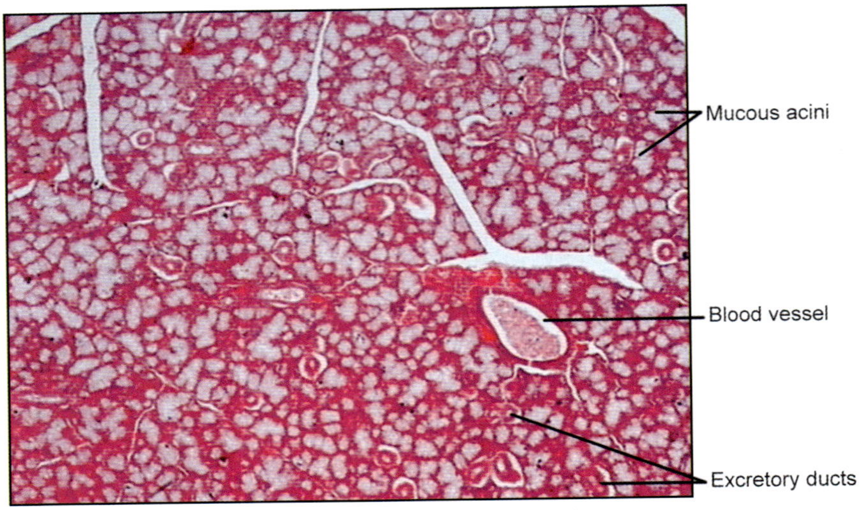

FIGURE 9.4 Mucous salivary gland, H & E, X40

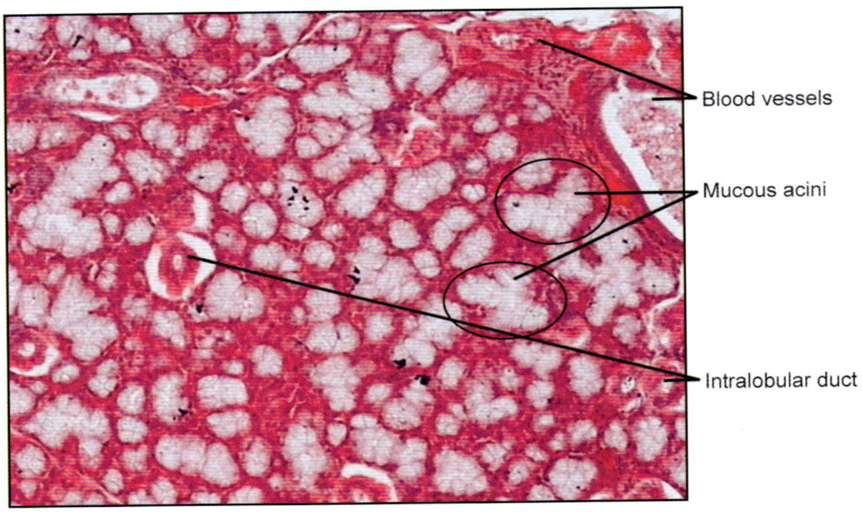

FIGURE 9.5 Mucous salivary gland, H & E, X100

MIXED SALIVARY GLAND

The submandibular is mixed gland with serous acini, mucous acini and serous demilunes. The serous acini predominates the gland.

Section under scanner (Fig. 9.7) reveals the mucous and serous acini. The excretory ducts are also seen. The ducts are lined by the columnar epithelium.

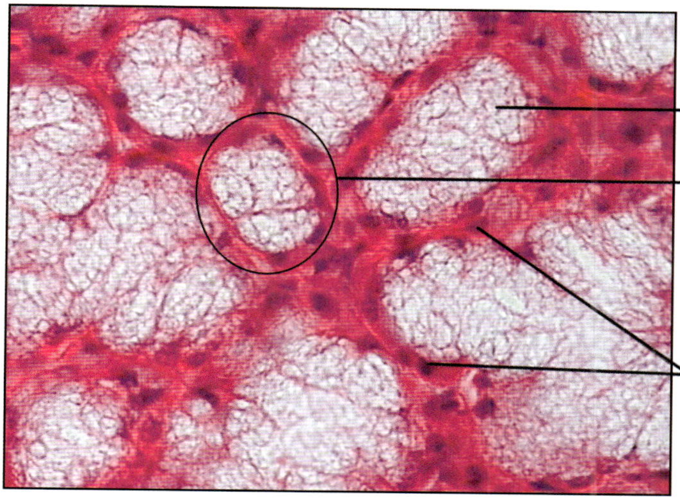

FIGURE 9.6 Mucous salivary gland, H & E, X400

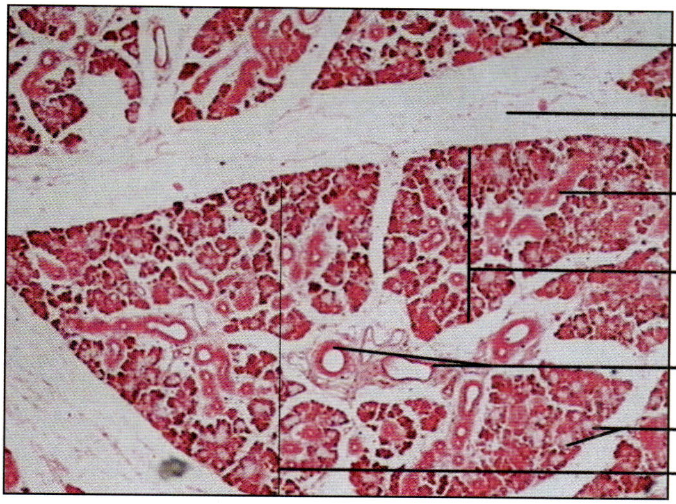

FIGURE 9.7 Mixed salivary gland, H & E, X40

The sections under low power (Fig. 9.8) and high power (Fig. 9.9) shows the serous mucous acini and serous demilune.

According to the recent evidence, the serous demilune is an artifact, in which the serous cells are squeezed out of their normal position by the swelling of the mucous cells. The excretory duct shows the striations formed from the infoldings of the cell membrane and mitochondria present between the infoldings. The myoepithelial cells present between the secretory cells and the basement membrane are difficult to locate in H & E preparation.

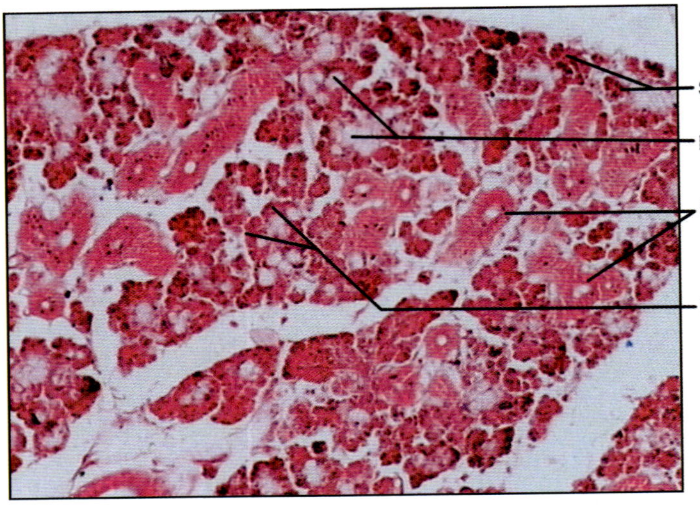

FIGURE 9.8 Mixed salivary gland, H & E, X100

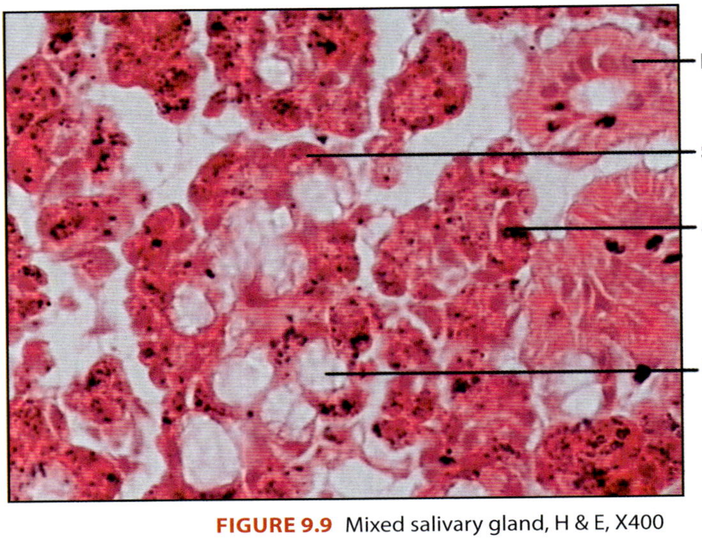

FIGURE 9.9 Mixed salivary gland, H & E, X400

POINTS TO REMEMBER

Types	*Serous*	*Mucous*	*Mixed*
Capsule	Connective tissue. Interlobular connective tissue with vessels and adipose tissue	Connective tissue. Well-developed connective tissue septa	Well-developed connective tissue capsule and stroma
Acini (alveoli)	Serous	Mucous	Seromucous
Cells	• Pyramidal in shape with round nuclei at the base. • Darkly stained apical cytoplasm because of the zymogen granules	• Globular in shape. Flat and condensed nuclei, at the basement membrane. • Cells appear empty in H and E staining, because mucinogen granules dissolved during processing. • Microvilli, pinocytotic vesicles and foldings of plasma membrane absent.	Both serous and mucous alveoli present. Demilunes or crescents of Giannuzzi, are the appearance of the sectioned serous alveoli seen as half moon or crescent shape over the mucous alveoli
Duct system-Intercalated (low cuboidal), Striated (simple cuboidal to columnar with basal infolding of cell membrane), interlobular/ interlobar (pseudostratified columnar/stratified cuboidal)	More, well developed intercalated, striated ducts	Few, short, poorly developed/absent intercalated, striated ducts	Short, few intercalated ducts and long striated ducts
Secretion	Watery secretion rich in enzymes and antibodies	Viscid secretion	Both watery as well as the viscid secretions
Example Salivary gland	Parotid	Sublingual	Submandibular

Note

Myoepithelial cells contractile in nature, present in the alveoli, intercalated ducts, large ducts of salivary glands, helping in secretion may be seen under high magnification. Under low power, the flat nuclei may be seen.

CHAPTER

10

Integumentary Tissue

Integumentary system includes skin, its derivatives and appendages. In human, skin derivatives are the nail, hair, several types of sweat and sebaceous glands. Skin consists of two layers; the superficial epidermis, which is nonvascular is lined by the keratinized stratified squamous epithelium and deeper dermis consisting of dense irregular connective tissue. Deep to the dermis is the hypodermis, the connective tissue layer and adipose tissue that forms the superficial fascia.

The histology of the skin is same all over the body, except the thickness in the epidermis. In palm and sole, epidermis is thick with the sweat glands, as the palm and sole are always exposed to increased wear, tear and abrasions. In the rest of the parts of the body, the skin is thin. The epidermis of the skin gives rise to nails, hair follicles, sebaceous glands and sweat glands. Attached to the connective tissue sheath of hair follicles and the connective tissue of dermis are the smooth muscle fibers, called the arrector pili. The epidermis grows continuously, but thickness remains the same, due to desquamation.

Dermis is the connective tissue layer and is highly vascular. Dermis gives mechanical support, strength and thickness to the skin. The junction of the dermis with epidermis is irregular. The superficial layer of dermis, the papillary layer forms raised projections, called the dermal papillae, interdigitating with the evaginations of epidermis, called the epidermal ridges. Dermis contains loose irregular connective tissue, connective tissue fibers, capillaries, blood vessels, fibroblasts, macrophages and other connective tissue cells.

The deeper reticular layer is thick and contains dense irregular connective tissue with connective tissue fibers and few cells.

Certain regions of skin consist of arteriovenous anastomoses for the temperature regulation, where blood passes directly from the arteries into the veins.

The hypodermis contains the superficial fascia and adipose tissue.

Section under scanner (Fig. 10.1) shows superficial and deep structures. The layers of the epidermis from superficial to deep layers are the stratum corneum, stratum lucidum stratum granulosum, stratum spinosum and stratum basale. Deep to the epidermis is the irregular dense connective tissue dermis. Dermal papilla and epidermal ridges are seen.

Section under low power (Fig. 10.2) shows the epidermis and dermis. The epidermis shows five layers. The surface shows dome-shaped contours representing the cross-section of the ridges, which produces the fingerprints characteristic to each individual. The dermis consists of sweat glands and blood vessels.

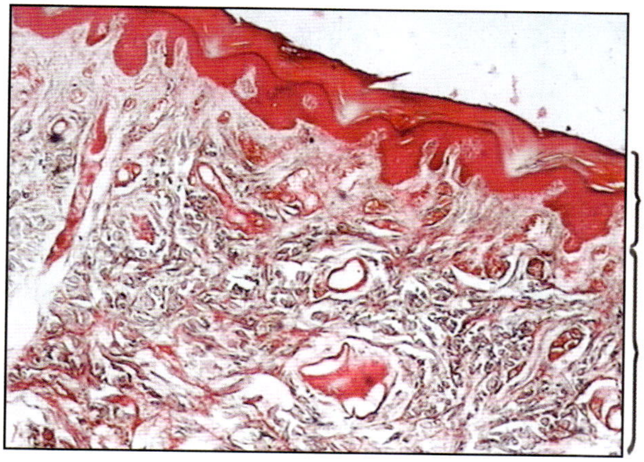

FIGURE 10.1 Thick skin, H & E, X40

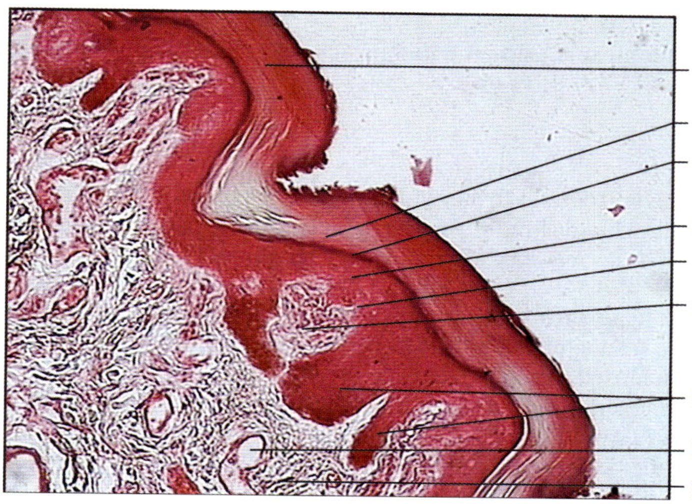

FIGURE 10.2 Thick skin, H & E, X100

Under the high power (Fig. 10.3), the section shows the five layers of epidermis, distinctly. The stratum corneum is a wide layer of flattened, dead, keratinized cells constantly being shed or desquamated from the surface of the skin. There is thin light stained stratum lucidum, which is difficult to see under the stratum corneum. Stratum lucidum has flattened cells and eleiden droplets.

Below stratum lucidum layer is the stratum granulosum, where the cells are filled with dark-stained keratohyalin granules. The thick layer, the stratum spinosum is composed of many layers of polyhedral cells and is present under the stratum granulosum. The adjacent cells in stratum spinosum layer are connected by spinous processes or intercellular bridge that represents the sites of desmosomes. The deepest layer stratum basale rests on the basement membrane. In stratum

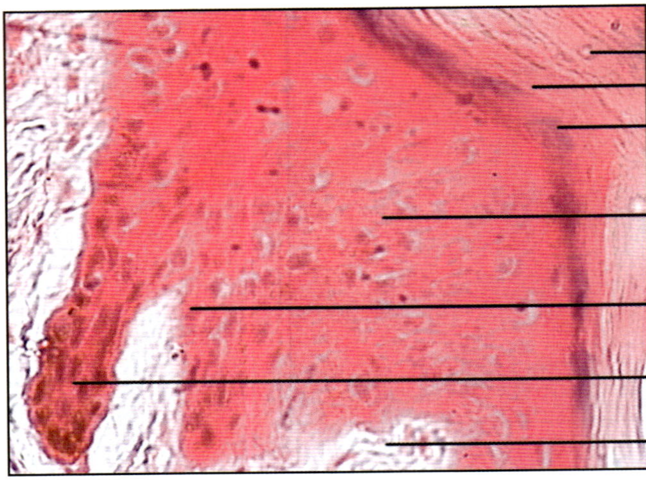

FIGURE 10.3 Thick skin, H & E, X400

basale and lower part of stratum spinosum, the mitotic activity and brown melanin pigment are seen.

THIN SKIN

Thin skin shows the epidermis and dermis. In the epidermis, stratum corneum, stratum granulosum, stratum spinosum, and stratum basale from superficial to deep layers respectively appreciated; but not the stratum lucidum. In the dermis, hair follicles, associated sebaceous glands and arrector pili muscle are seen.

Section under scanner (Fig. 10.4) shows the epidermis and dermis. The layers of epidermis are difficult to be identified. The section of hair follicle, sebaceous gland opening into the hair follicle, sweat gland and arrector pili muscle are seen.

Section under low power (Fig. 10.5) shows the section of hair follicle, associated sebaceous gland, arrector pili muscle and sweat glands.

In the section is shown the different parts of the hair follicle. From outside inwards, the layers present are—connective tissue sheath, outer root sheath, inner root sheath and cuticle. The root of hair and dermal papilla (dermis invaginating into root of hair) together form hair bulb. Here outer and inner root sheaths merge into hair matrix (undifferentiated cells).

Adjacent to the hair follicle in the connective tissue of dermis, sebaceous glands and arrector pili muscle are shown. The sebaceous gland and the arrector pili are always associated with the hair follicle. The sebaceous gland is lined with a stratified epithelium, which continues with the external root sheath of the hair follicle. The base is lined by columnar or cuboidal cells, called the basal cells resting on basement membrane. Basal cells divide and fill the gland with large polyhedral secretory cells. The secretory cells in the center of the acinus undergo degeneration and become oily secretory product, the sebum, which passes to the lumen of the hair follicle through short ducts. The arrector pili muscle when contracts force the sebum out of the sebaceous gland and make the hair follicle to stand up forming dimple or goose bump on the skin. The sweat gland consists of two types of epithelial cells (dark and clear) and myoepithelial cells. Dark cells are close to the lumen and clear cells are related to the base of the epithelial layer making contact with the basal lamina or myoepithelial cells.

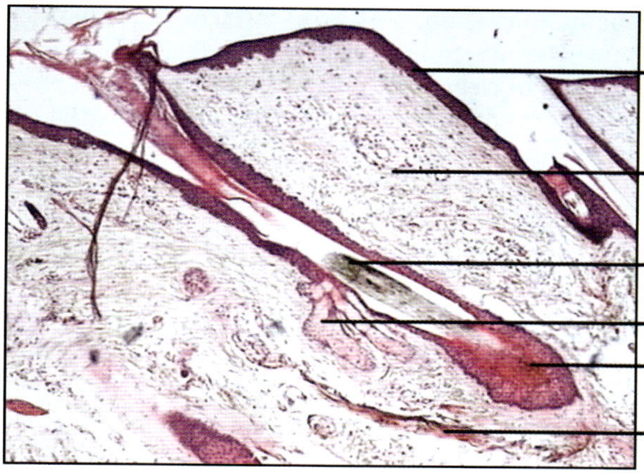

FIGURE 10.4 Thin skin, H & E, X40

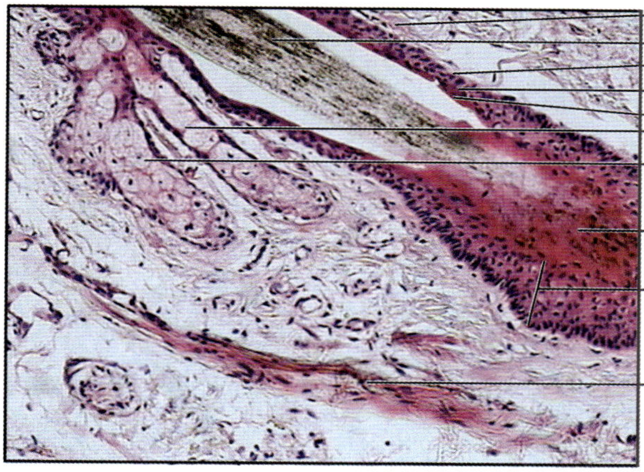

FIGURE 10.5 Thin skin, H & E, X100

POINTS TO REMEMBER

Thick Skin

Epidermis: Stratified squamous keratinized epithelium (four types of cells: keratinocytes, melanocytes, Langerhans' cells, Merkel's cells) and 5 layers of strata from the dermis to the surface.

- *Stratum basale (stratum germinativum):* Basophilic columnar or cuboidal cells separate dermis from epidermis and characterized by intense mitotic activity.
- *Stratum spinosum:* Named because of the prickly appearance of the cells. Cells are in the processes of growth and early keratin synthesis.
- *Stratum granulosum:* 2–5 rows of flattened rhombic-shaped cells, long-axis parallel to the surface of skin and with numerous coarse basophilic keratohyaline granules.

- *Stratum lucidum:* More apparent in thick skin. Few rows of flattened cells, appears as homogeneous translucent band and contain semifluid droplets called eleidin.
- *Stratum corneum:* Very thick composed of clear, dead scale-like cells and cells become more and more flattened nearer to the surface with fine filamentous fibrous protein, the keratin.
- *Apart from the keratinocytes is the presence of 3 other cell types:* Melanocytes, Langerhans cells and Merkel cells.

Dermis: Varies from 0.2 mm to 4 mm in thickness.

- Composed of irregularly arranged connective tissue with three types of fibers (collagen, elastic and reticular), fibroblasts and other connective tissue cells.
- 2 layers distinguished are the deeper reticular and superficial papillary layers.
- A rich network of blood and lymph vessels and sweat glands is present.
- Hair follicles, sebaceous glands and arrector pili muscles are absent.
- *For example:* Palm, sole, some parts of male and female external genitalia.

Thin Skin

Epidermis: Structure is similar to that of the thick skin, except that the stratum lucidum is absent and the other layers are thin when compared to the thick skin.

Dermis: Structure similar to thick skin except for the presence of hair follicles, sweat glands, sebaceous glands and arrector pili muscle.

Appendages

Hair follicle: Three layers from within outwards:

1. *Inner root sheath:* Only in lower part of follicle with three layers:
   a. *Inner most layer:* Cuticle: Flattened cornified cells.
   b. *Huxley's layer:* Flattened nucleated cells with eosinophilic granules.
   c. *Henley's layer:* Cubical cells with flattened nuclei.
2. *Outer root sheath:* Living, rounded, nucleated cells. Below the sheath is continued with the hair bulb and above with the stratum spinosum of skin.
3. *Connective tissue sheath:* Highly vascular, numerous nerve fibers, continuous with dermis.

Sweat glands: Widely distributed in the skin.

- Merocrine, simple, coiled, tubular glands embedded in the dermis surrounded by myoepithelial cells.
- Secretory portion has two types of cells, the dark and the clear cells.
- Ducts lined with stratified cuboidal epithelium, open onto the surface of the skin.
- Secrete nonviscous fluid.

Sebaceous glands:

- Holocrine, simple or branched acinar glands.
- Both the acini and ducts lined with stratified squamous epithelium.
- Ducts are wide, usually open in the upper portion of the hair follicle, but in some regions (glans penis, clitoris, lips, nipple) open directly onto the epidermal surface.
- Secretes sebum.

Arrector pili muscle:

- Smooth muscle in obtuse angle between the hair follicles and the surface of the skin.
- Contractions promote erection of the hair shaft into vertical position (goose flesh).
- For example, scalp, rest of the body.

CHAPTER

11

Respiratory System

The respiratory system consists of lungs and numerous air passages or tubes of various sizes. It has conducting portion (extrapulmonary—tachea, primary bronchi; intrapulmonary—secondary bronchi, bronchioles), transition zone (respiratory bronchioles) and respiratory portion (alveolar ducts, alveolar sacs, alveoli). The conducting portion conducts air for gaseous exchange to and from the lungs, the transition zone is involved both in air conduction and gas exchange and the respiratory portion allows respiration or gaseous exchange.

The extrapulmonary and intrapulmonary passages are lined by pseudostratified ciliated columnar epithelium with numerous goblet cells. Towards the bronchioles, the diameters become smaller, lining epithelium decreases in height, amount of cilia and numbers of goblet cells also decrease. In alveoli, the goblet cells are absent and the epithelium is simple squamous.

TRACHEA

Trachea is a short tube of about 2.5 cm in diameter and extends about 10 cm in length. It extends from the larynx to the middle of the thorax, where it divides into the two primary bronchi. Its major function is to conduct the air. The lumen is held open by numerous C-shaped hyaline cartilages arranged on one another to form a supporting structure. Fibroblastic tissue and smooth muscle, the trachealis muscle, fill the gap between the free ends of the cartilages, at the posterior part of the trachea, adjacent to the esophagus. Typical respiratory epithelium (ciliated pseudostratified columnar) lines the trachea and primary bronchi.

The section under scanner (Fig. 11.1) shows the mucosa, submucosa, hyaline cartilage (Fibromusculocartilaginous layer) and adventitia. Mucosa has epithelial layer (pseudostratified ciliated columnar epithelium with goblet cells), lamina propria (fine connective tissue fibers, diffuse lymphatic tissue, occasional solitary lymphatic nodules) and longitudinal elastic membrane, which divides the lamina propria from the submucosa. The submucosa has loose connective tissue and tubuloacinar seromucous tracheal glands. Along the posterior wall of the trachea, the mucosa is thrown into folds, hyaline cartilage is absent and the glands in submucosa may extend into the adventitia.

Next to submucosa is the C-shaped hyaline cartilage surrounded by perichondrium that merges with the submucosa on the luminal side and the adventitia on the other side. The gap between the posterior ends of cartilage is filled by smooth muscle, the trachealis muscle attached to

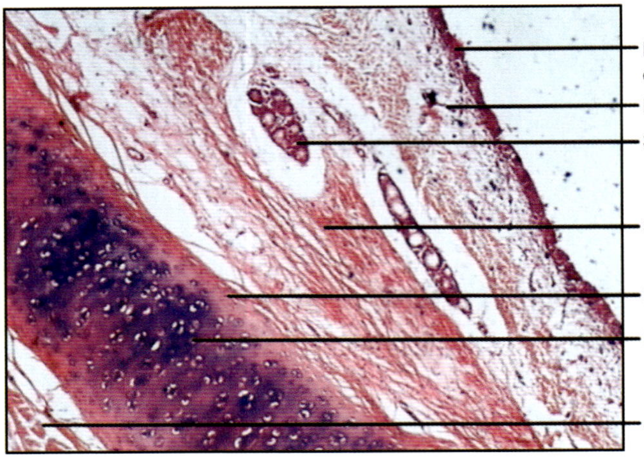

FIGURE 11.1 Trachea, H & E, X40

the perichondrium. Covering the hyaline cartilage is the adventitia with numerous nerves, blood vessels and adipose tissue.

Section under low power (Fig. 11.2) shows the mucosa and submucosa. The pseudostratified ciliated columnar epithelium has few goblet cells. The basement membrane is not very clear. The lamina propria is cellular in nature and the elastic membrane and submucosa are clearly observed. Seromucous glands are evident in the submucosa.

Section under high power (Fig. 11.3) shows the epithelial layer, the cilia of the pseudostratified ciliated columnar epithelium and the dense line formed by the basal bodies of the cilia in the apical cytoplasm. Goblet cells are observed and the displacement of the flattened nuclei toward the base of the cells is well-demonstrated.

LUNG

Lungs are made up of alveoli or air sacs facilitating the exchange of gases, a system of intrapulmonary air passages (secondary and tertiary bronchi, bronchioles, terminal bronchioles, respiratory bronchioles, alveolar ducts, alveolar sacs) and rich capillary network supported by elastic connective tissue.

The lungs have dual blood supply, the pulmonary system and the bronchial system. The pulmonary supply carries deoxygenated blood from the right side of the heart via large pulmonary artery to each lung.

The pulmonary arteries enter the roots or hila of the lungs, with the main bronchi and then divide and course parallel to the branching airways to supply the pulmonary capillaries, surrounding the alveoli. The pulmonary arterial system is structurally unusual in two respects. Firstly, the pulmonary arterial vessels are relatively thin-walled and of large caliber, their diameter approximating that of the accompanying airway. The arterial blood pressure in the pulmonary arterial system is much lower than the systemic blood pressure. Secondly, the pulmonary arteries have the histological characteristics of elastic arteries rather than of muscular arteries. Elastic expansion and recoil of the vessels maintain the pulmonary arterial pressure at a relatively constant level, throughout the cardiac cycle.

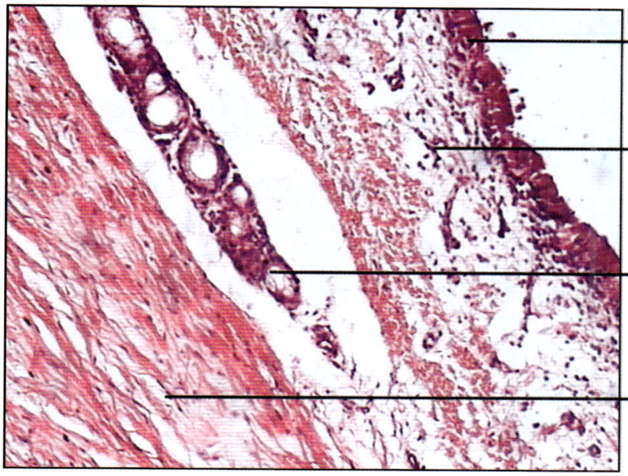

FIGURE 11.2 Trachea, H & E, X100

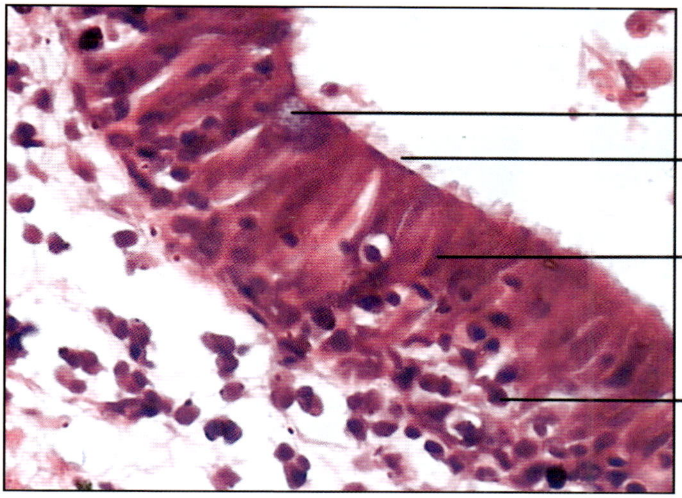

FIGURE 11.3 Trachea, H & E, X400

The bronchial arterial system constitutes the systemic circulation of the lower respiratory tract. It arises as small branches of the aorta and supplies oxygenated blood to the tissues of the airway walls and to the pleura, the layer that invests the outer surface of each lung. The bronchial vessels are of the usual type found in the rest of the systemic circulation.

A common venous system returns most of the blood to the left side of the heart via the pulmonary veins of thin-walled vessels of wide diameter. A small proportion of blood from the bronchial system drains to the right side of the heart via the azygous venous system.

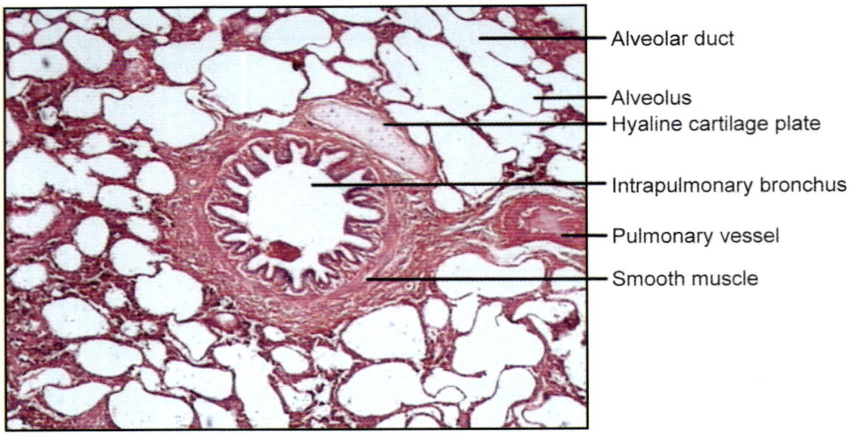

FIGURE 11.4A Lung, H & E, X40

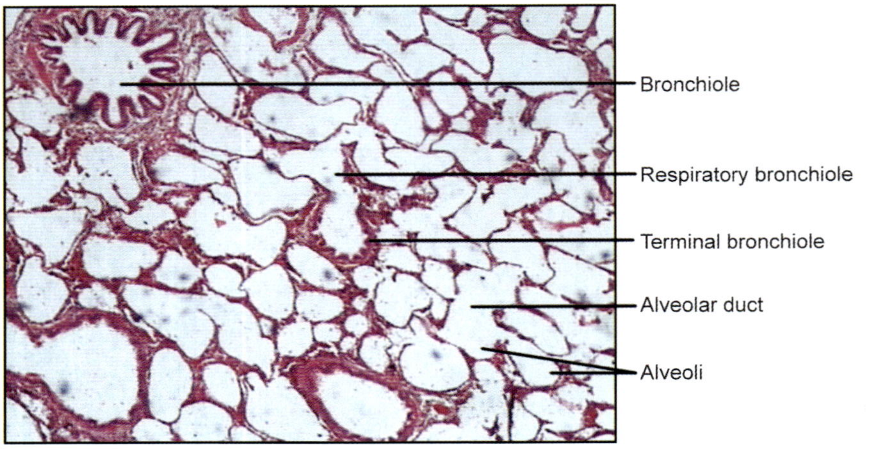

FIGURE 11.4B Lung, H & E, X40

The sections under scanner (Figs 11.4A and B) show the intrapulmonary bronchi, bronchioles and alveoli. The intrapulmonary bronchi divide to form the bronchioles that in turn subdivide into the smaller terminal bronchioles, the diameters of which are approximately 1 mm or less. The bronchi are lined by pseudostratified ciliated columnar epithelium with layers of smooth muscle and irregular hyaline cartilage plates. The terminal bronchioles, the epithelium may be simple cuboidal. The cartilage plates, bronchial glands and goblet cells are absent in the terminal bronchiole. The terminal bronchiole represents the smallest passageways for conducting the air.

Because of smooth muscle contractions, mucosal folds are prominent in the bronchioles. A well-developed smooth muscle layer surrounds the thin lamina propria, that in turn is surrounded by the adventitia.

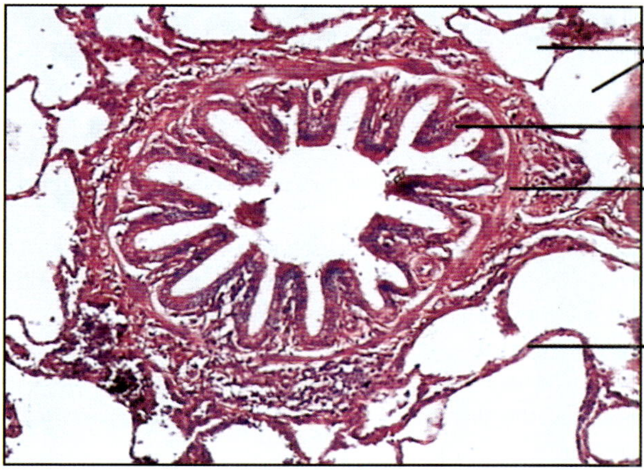

FIGURE 11.5 Lung, H & E, X100

Adjacent to the bronchi are the small branches of the pulmonary artery. The bronchi and terminal bronchiole are surrounded by the lung alveoli. Alveoli are lined by type 1 and type 2 pneumocytes and surrounded by thin interalveolar septa with capillaries.

Section under low power (Fig. 11.5) shows the terminal bronchioles giving rise to the respiratory bronchioles representing the transition zone between the conducting and respiratory portions of the respiratory system. The wall of the respiratory bronchiole is lined by the simple cuboidal epithelium. Single alveolar pocketings are found in the wall of each respiratory bronchiole. Cilia may be present in the epithelium of the proximal portion of the respiratory bronchiole, but disappear in the distal portion. A thin layer of smooth muscle surrounds the epithelium. A small branch of the pulmonary artery accompanies the respiratory bronchiole into the lung. Each respiratory bronchiole gives rise to an alveolar duct into which open numerous alveoli. In the lamina propria, that surrounds the rim of alveoli in the alveolar duct are the smooth muscle bundles, which appear as knobs between the adjacent alveoli.

The alveoli are evaginations or outpocketings of the respiratory bronchioles, alveolar ducts and alveolar sacs, the terminal ends of the alveolar ducts. A layer of thin simple squamous alveolar cells, fine connective tissue fibers with fibroblasts and numerous capillaries line the alveoli. The thin interalveolar septa bring the capillaries close to the squamous alveolar cells of the adjacent alveoli.

In addition, the alveoli also contain alveolar macrophages. Normally, the alveolar macrophages contain several carbon or dust particles in their cytoplasm. Also found in the alveoli, are the great alveolar cells, type II pneumocytes. The great alveolar cells in the alveoli are interspersed among the simple squamous alveolar macrophages.

At the free ends of the interalveolar septa and around the open ends of the alveoli are the narrow bands of smooth muscle fibers, which continue with the muscle layer lining the respiratory bronchioles.

POINTS TO REMEMBER

Trachea

Mucosa	
• Epithelium	Tall, pseudostratified columnar ciliated epithelium and goblet cells rich with mucinogen granules
• Lamina propria	Loose, highly vascular connective tissue condensed at deeper aspects to form a fibroelastic tissue
Submucosa	Loose connective tissue with numerous seromucous glands
Fibromusculo-cartilaginous layer	Deep to the lamina propria, C- shaped hyaline cartilage and fibrous tissue with the smooth muscle, the trachealis attached to the ends of the cartilage in the posterior part
Adventitia	Surrounds fibromusculocartilaginous ring. Consists of connective tissue with large blood vessels, nerves and lymphatics

Cells in Respiratory Passage

- Pseudostratified ciliated columnar cells
- Goblet cells (mucous)
- Nonciliated columnar cells (serous)
- Clara cells (surfactant)
- Kulchitsky cells (hormones/serotonin)
- Basal cells (reserve cells)
  - Type 1 alveolar cell (gaseous exchange)
  - Type 2 alveolar cells (surfactant)
  - Macrophages/Dust cells (remove inhaled particulate matter).

Lung

- Honeycomb appearance of the alveoli
- Alveoli lined by squamous cells
- Divisions of bronchial tree from the intrapulmonary bronchi to the terminal bronchiole
- Respiratory unit
- Pulmonary vessels accompanying bronchioles.

Additional Information

- *Respiratory bronchiole*
  - Regions of transitions between the conducting and respiratory portions.
  - Lined by simple ciliated cuboidal epithelium.
  - Walls interrupted by numerous saccular alveoli which continue with the squamous epithelium.
  - Smooth muscle layer and elastic connective tissue overlie the epithelium.
- *Alveolar duct*
  - Lined by simple squamous epithelium.
  - Smooth muscle layer with elastic and collagen fibrils, support the epithelium.

- *Atria/ alveolar sac*
  - Lined by squamous epithelium
  - Numerous elastic and reticular fibers encircle the epithelium.
- *Alveoli*
  - The evaginations of respiratory bronchioles, alveolar ducts and alveolar sacs.
  - Two thin squamous epithelial layers between which lie capillaries, elastic fibers, collagen fibers and fibroblasts.
  - Walls composed of three main cell types:
    1. Type I pneumocytes (squamous)
    2. Type II pneumocytes (septal or great alveolar or surfactant cells)
    3. Macrophages (dust cells, heart failure cells).
- Blood- air barrier composition:
  - Surfactant.
  - Alveolar epithelium.
  - Basal lamina of alveolar epithelium.
  - Basal lamina of capillary endothelium.
  - Capillary endothelium.

DIFFERENCES BETWEEN THE PARTS OF BRONCHIAL TREE

Parts	*Epithelium*	*Features of wall*
Trachea	Pseudostratified ciliated columnar epithelium, goblet cells, brush cells (nonciliated columnar), Kulchitsky cells (small granule cells), basal cells	Lamina propria, submucosa with seromucous glands, fibromusculocartilaginous layer, adventitia
Bronchi	Pseudostratified ciliated columnar epithelium with goblet cells	Narrow thin lamina propria, layer of smooth muscle cells, submucosa with bronchial glands, irregular hyaline cartilage plates, adventitia
Bronchiole	Pseudostratified ciliated columnar to simple cuboidal epithelium from proximal to distal with occasional goblet cells	Mucosal folds, smooth muscle layer, adventitia. No cartilage and glands
Terminal bronchiole	Simple cuboidal epithelium, clara cells	Thin, incomplete layer of smooth muscle. No cartilage and glands
Respiratory bronchiole	Simple cuboidal epithelium, clara cells with scattered alveoli	Few smooth muscle fibers mostly around alveolar openings
Alveolar ducts, sacs	Simple cuboidal between many alveoli	Bands of smooth muscle around alveolar openings
Alveoli	Type 1 and type 2 alveolar cells (pneumocytes)	Only network of elastic and reticular fibers

CHAPTER

12

Digestive System

The digestive system is a long, hollow tube starting from the oral cavity to the anus. The parts of the digestive system are oral cavity, esophagus, stomach, small intestine, large intestine, rectum and anal canal. The accessory digestive organs associated with the digestive system are the salivary glands, liver and pancreas and excretory ducts connect the glands to the small intestine.

The mucosa of the digestive system performs numerous functions like secretion (digestive enzymes, hydrochloric acid, mucin, antibodies), absorption (metabolic substrates: breakdown products of digestion, vitamins, water, electrolytes, recyclable materials like bile and cholesterol, substances essential for body functions), barrier (entry of noxious substances, antigens, pathogenic organisms) and immunologic protection (lymphatic tissue in mucosa acts as the first line of immune defense).

TONGUE

Tongue is a muscular organ in the oral cavity. The tongue is covered with mucous membrane lined by the partly keratinized stratified squamous epithelium. The core of the tongue consists of connective tissue and interlacing bundles of skeletal muscle fibers. The increased movements during chewing, swallowing and speaking are because of the random distribution of individual skeletal muscle fibers.

The epithelium of the tongue is smooth on the ventral surface and rough on the dorsal surface, because of the projections, called the papillae. The anterior 2/3rd of the dorsal surface of the tongue has the papillae covered by the stratified squamous epithelium with partial or incomplete keratinization. The posterior 1/3rd of the tongue contains lymph follicles and lingual tonsils and lined by nonkeratinized stratified squamous epithelium. The four types of papillae are the filiform, fungiform, circumvallate and foliate. Foliate is not seen in human. The papillae appear as red dots when examined macroscopically.

Among the papillae, filiform papillae are more numerous and cover the entire dorsal surface of the tongue. Fungiform papillae are broad with nonkeratinized epithelium and are less numerous present at the sides and tip of tongue. Circumvallate papillae are seven to twelve in number arranged in V-shaped manner, at the junction of the anterior 2/3rd (body) and posterior 1/3rd of the tongue (root).

Deep to the epithelium and papillae is the lamina propria with loose connective tissue, numerous blood vessels and nerve fibers. The core of the tongue deep to lamina propria consists of the interlacing bundles of skeletal muscle arranged in longitudinal and transverse planes.

Section under scanner (Fig. 12.1) shows the filiform and the fungiform papillae. Deep to the surface are the lamina propria and the bulk of the skeletal muscle fibers. Connective tissue and blood vessels are in the lamina propria.

Section under low power (Fig. 12.2) shows the filiform papillae. The filiform papillae are the bent sharp conical projections of the epithelium directed posteriorly. Taste buds are absent in filiform papillae. Filiform papillae covered by the stratified squamous epithelium show partial keratinization over the tip.

Section under low power (Fig. 12.3) shows mushroom-like larger, taller and broader fungiform papillae. The fungiform papillae are prevalent in the anterior part of the tongue, less numerous and

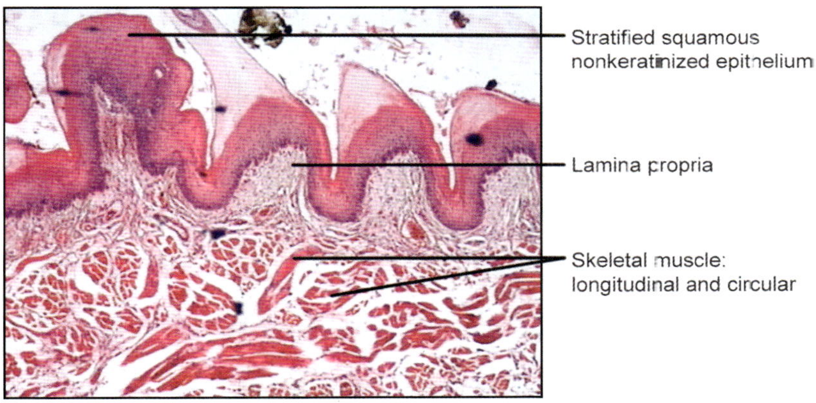

FIGURE 12.1 Tongue, H & E, X40

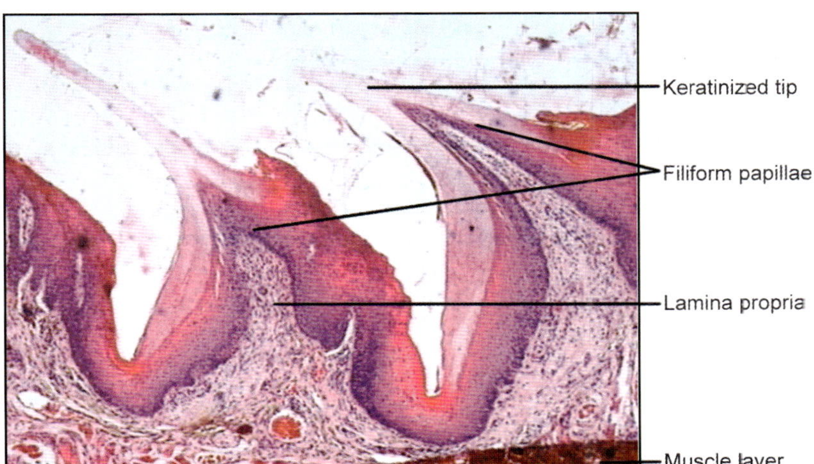

FIGURE 12.2 Tongue, filiform papillae, H & E, X100

are interspersed between the filiform papillae. Fungiform papillae have nonkeratinized stratified squamous epithelium and a core of lamina propria. In the epithelium towards the surface, few taste buds may be present. Small connective tissue papillae project into the epithelium.

Section under scanner and low power (Figs 12.4 and 12.5) shows the circumvallate papillae. The circumvallate papillae are surrounded by the deep trench or furrow and covered by the nonkeratinized stratified squamous epithelium with a core of lamina propria. The lamina propria exhibits numerous secondary papillae projecting into the epithelium. The lateral surfaces of the circumvallate papillae have the oval taste buds. Numerous tubuloacinar serous or von Ebner's glands opening into the bottom of the trench are present in the lamina propria and core of the tongue.

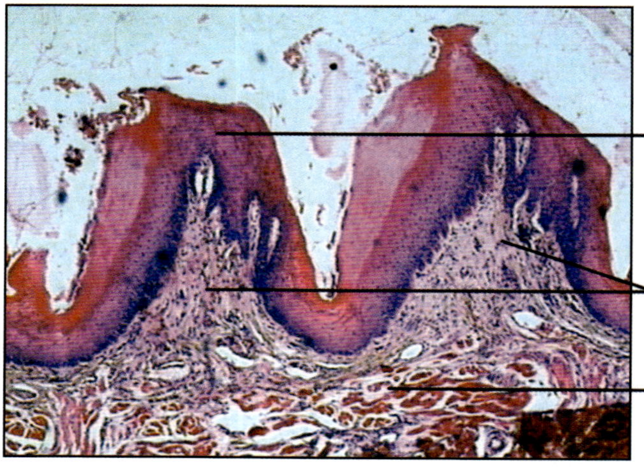

FIGURE 12.3 Tongue, fungiform papillae, H & E, X100

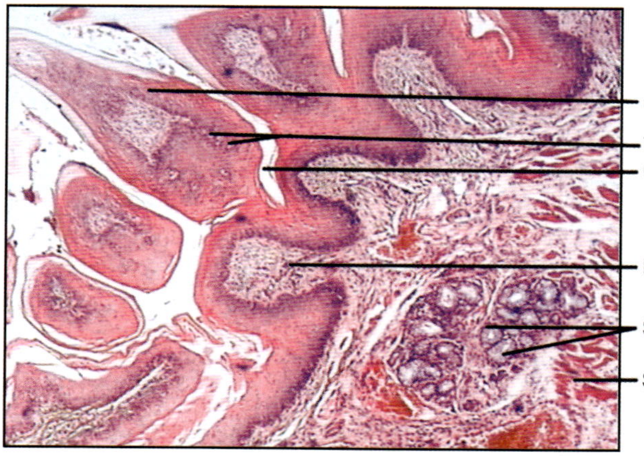

FIGURE 12.4 Tongue, circumvallate papillae, H & E, X40

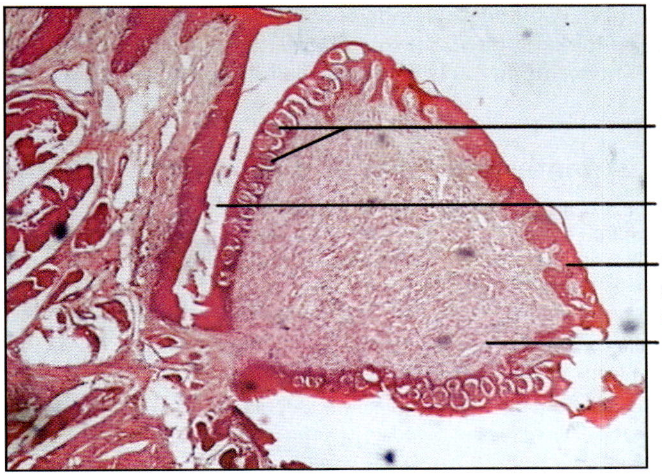

FIGURE 12.5 Tongue, circumvallate papillae, H & E, X100

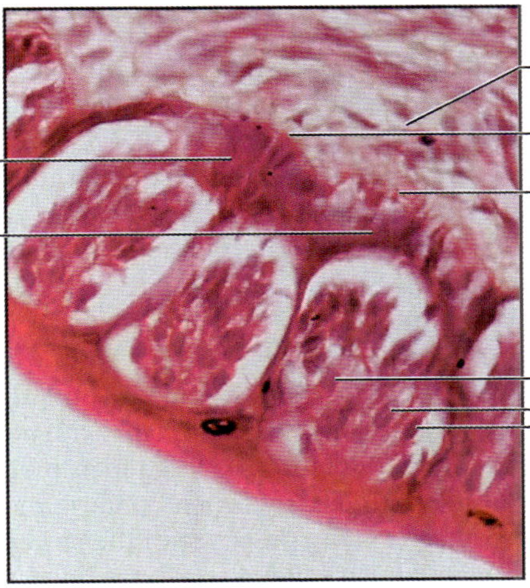

FIGURE 12.6 Taste buds, H & E, X400

Section under high power (Fig. 12.6) shows the taste buds. The taste buds occupy the whole thickness of the epithelium in the lateral wall of the circumvallate papillae and also are present in the surface epithelium of the fungiform papillae. The taste buds are oval in shape and elongated and are modified columnar cells arranged perpendicular to the epithelium and open at the surface through a small pore. Three types of cells are present in the taste buds. Sustentacular cells or supporting cells are elongated and show dark cytoplasm and slender dark nucleus. The gustatory cells or taste cells or sensory cells or neuroepithelial cells show lighter cytoplasm and oval lighter nucleus. The basal cells are present at the periphery of the taste buds near the basement membrane. Taste pore, a small opening is towards the epithelial surface. Sensory fibers ending within the taste buds are the intragemmal fibers and some fibers ending freely in the epithelium in between the taste buds are the intergemmal fibers.

General Structure of Gastrointestinal Tract from Esophagus to Rectum

Mucous membrane	Epithelium—varies. Lamina propria—connective tissue with blood and lymph vessels, lymphatic tissue, glands and smooth muscle cells Muscularis mucosae—inner circular and outer longitudinal smooth muscle layers
Submucosa	Irregular connective tissue with large blood vessels, lymphatic vessels, Meissner's nerve plexus, glands and lymphatic tissue in some parts
Muscularis externa	Inner circular and outer longitudinal smooth muscle layers with myenteric (Auerbach's) nerve plexus, blood and lymph vessels
Serosa	Loose connective tissue with blood and lymph vessels covered by flattened epithelium, the mesothelium

ESOPHAGUS

Esophagus a hollow, muscular tube, 10 inches in length, extends from the pharynx to the stomach. The wall of the esophagus consists of mucosa, submucosa, muscularis externa and adventitia from within outwards.

The mucosa has three layers, inner epithelial layer of nonkeratinized stratified squamous epithelium, middle thin layer of fine connective tissue lamina propria and a layer of longitudinal smooth muscle fibers, the muscularis mucosae. The connective tissue in the lamina propria indent the epithelium to form the connective tissue papillae and it has small blood vessels, diffuse lymphatic tissue and small lymphatic nodule.

The submucosa is wide with moderately dense irregular connective tissue and often has adipose tissue. The esophageal glands, numerous blood vessels, lymphatic vessels and submucosal or Meissner's plexus are present in the submucosa. The excretory ducts of the esophageal glands pass through the muscularis mucosae and lamina propria to open into the lumen.

The muscularis externa is composed of inner circular and outer longitudinal muscle layers. In human, in the upper third of the esophagus is the presence of the striated skeletal muscle, in the middle third it is both smooth and skeletal muscle fibers and in the lower third only smooth muscle fibers are present. In between the two layers of muscle fibers is a thin connective tissue layer with myenteric plexus (Auerbach's plexus).

The adventitia has loose connective tissue, adipose tissue, large blood vessels and nerve fibers. The esophagus is surrounded only by connective tissue in the thoracic cavity, hence called adventitia, but in the abdominal cavity it is called serosa, since it is lined by the peritoneum. Peritoneum has simple squamous epithelium known as the mesothelium and small amount of underlying connective tissue.

Under the section of scanner (Fig. 12.7) the mucosa and submucosa are identified. The three layers of mucosa (nonkeratinized stratified squamous epithelium; lamina propria with blood vessels, nerves and lymphatics; muscularis mucosa) are evident. The connective tissue papillae of the lamina propria are identified. The submucosa with mucous type of esophageal glands is visible.

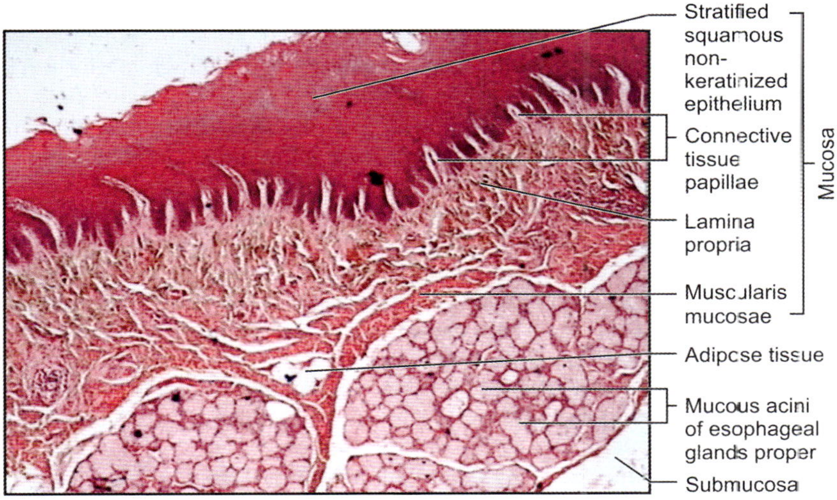

FIGURE 12.7 Esophagus, H & E, X40

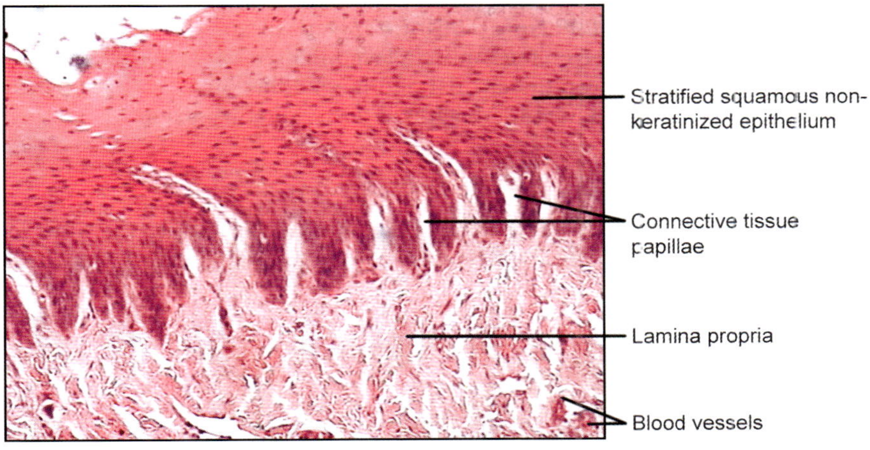

FIGURE 12.8 Esophagus, H & E, X100

Section under low power (Fig. 12.8) shows the nonkeratinized stratified squamous epithelium and lamina propria. In the epithelium the shape and orientation of the cells change as they migrate from basal layer to superficial layers. The nuclei are spherical in the deeper layers and in the superficial layers are elongated and oriented parallel to the surface. The nuclei are present throughout the epithelium especially in the superficial layers and the section shows that the epithelium is not keratinized.

Lamina propria is very cellular with loose connective tissue and blood vessels.

STOMACH

Stomach is the expanded muscular organ located beneath the diaphragm performing numerous functions. The stomach receives, stores, mixes and digests ingested food products and secretes hormones that regulate digestive functions. Stomach is divided into three parts—the cardia, fundus and body, and pylorus. The wall of the stomach consists of four layers, the mucosa, submucosa, muscularis externa and serosa.

The surface of the stomach is lined by simple columnar epithelium, which extends into and lines the gastric pits. The gastric pits are the tubular infoldings of surface epithelium, which are not deep. The pits extend 1/4th of the thickness of mucosa in the fundus, but are deep in the pylorus.

The lamina propria fills the spaces between the gastric glands. Gastric glands occupies the entire length of the lamina propria and open into the bottom of the gastric pits. There are four types of cells: Pale staining mucous neck cells, eosinophilic parietal cells, basophilic zymogenic (chief) cells and enteroendocrine cells. Parietal cells occupy the upper part and chief cells occupy the lower part of the gastric glands. There may be small lymphatic tissue or nodules in the subglandular regions of the lamina propria.

Muscularis mucosa has inner circular and outer longitudinal layers.

In the empty stomach, the mucosa forms temporary folds, the rugae, which disappears as the stomach fills and distends.

The submucosa in the empty stomach enters the rugae. The submucosa contains dense irregular connective tissue, more collagen fibers, lymph vessels, capillaries, arterioles, venules and clusters of parasympathetic ganglia of submucosal (Meissner's) nerve plexus.

Muscularis externa has inner oblique muscle layer, middle circular muscle layer and outer longitudinal muscle layer. Between the circular and longitudinal muscle layers parasympathetic ganglia and nerve fibers of myenteric (Auerbach's) nerve plexus are present.

Stomach Fundus

Section under scanner (Fig. 12.9) shows mucosa, submucosa and rugae. The three layers of the mucosa are visible. The luminal surface is lined by simple columnar epithelium which continues

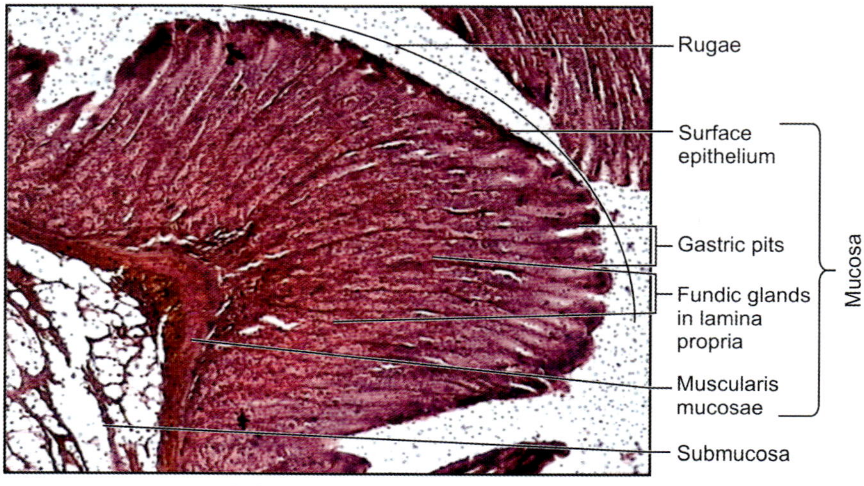

FIGURE 12.9 Stomach fundus, H & E, X40

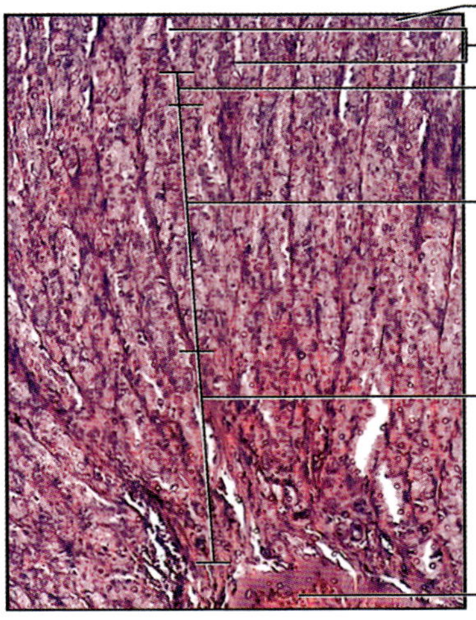

FIGURE 12.10 Stomach, fundus, H & E, X100

with the shallow gastric pits. The lamina propria has fibroblasts, lymphoid tissue, lymphocytes and other loose connective tissue cells and is better seen in mucosal ridges. The gastric glands extend throughout the lamina propria and open into the gastric pits. In the deeper regions of the mucosa the glands branch and appear as transverse and oblique sections. The submucosa is formed by dense connective tissue, collagen fibers, nuclei of fibroblasts, arterioles, venules, lymphatics, capillaries and adipose cells.

Section under low power (Fig. 12.10) shows the parts of the gastric glands. Isthmus is present at the junction of the gastric pits and gastric glands and is lined by surface epithelial cells and parietal cells. Neck present in the lower part of the isthmus contains mainly mucous neck cells and some parietal cells. The base or fundus present in the deep portion of the gland contains predominantly chief cells, few enteroendocrine cells and few parietal cells. The parietal and chief cells are properly visible in the section.

Section under high power (Fig. 12.11) shows the cells of the gastric glands. The mucous neck cells have round, basal nuclei and are located just below the gastric pits interspersed between the parietal cells. The parietal cells are large, polygonal, pyramidal shape with round nuclei and eosinophilic cytoplasm. The free surfaces of the parietal cells open into the gastric glands and secrete hydrochloric acid, gastric intrinsic factor necessary for the absorption of vitamin B_{12}. The chief cells are cuboidal and stain basophilic. The chief cells contain secretory granules that contain pepsinogen. Enteroendocrine cells secrete variety of polypeptides and proteins.

Stomach Pylorus

Section under scanner (Fig. 12.12) shows mucosa, submucosa, muscularis externa and serosa. The three layers of the mucosa are visible. The luminal surface is lined by simple columnar epithelium which continues with the deep gastric pits. The lamina propria has fibroblasts, lymphoid tissue, lymphocytes and other loose connective tissue cells. The pyloric glands extend throughout the lamina propria and open into the bottom of gastric pits. The pyloric glands are branched or coiled tubular glands containing mucous secretions. Compared to the fundic glands, the pyloric glands

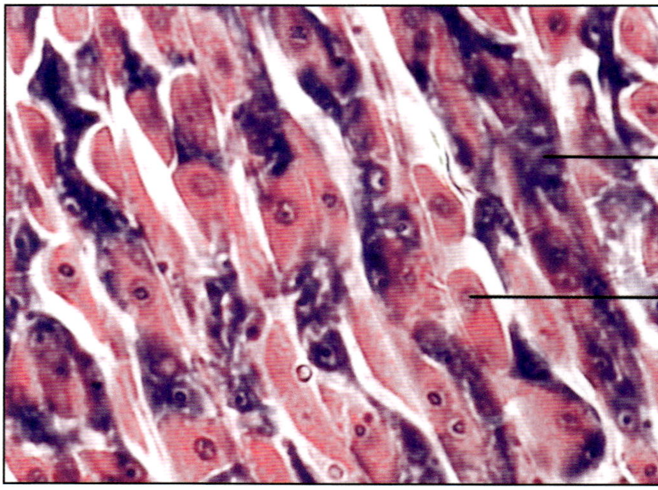

FIGURE 12.11 Stomach fundus, H & E, X400

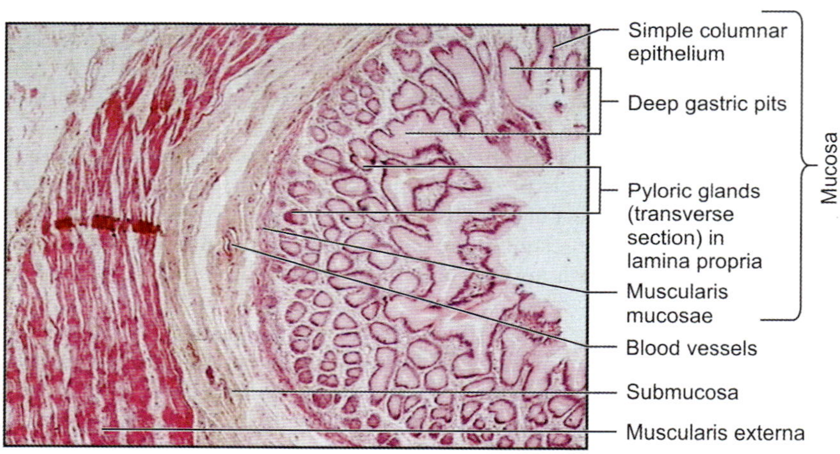

FIGURE 12.12 Stomach pylorus, H & E, X40

have longer pits and shorter coiled secretory part. The muscularis mucosa is seen deep to the lamina propria. The submucosa is irregular connective tissue with arterioles and venules. The muscularis externa is composed of smooth muscle cells arranged in outer longitudinal, middle circular and inner oblique layers. The serosa is seen outer to the muscularis externa.

The section under low power (Fig. 12.13) shows the mucosa and submucosa. The pyloric glands opening into the deep gastric pits are observed. In the lamina propria numerous transverse sections of coiled tubular pyloric glands are seen.

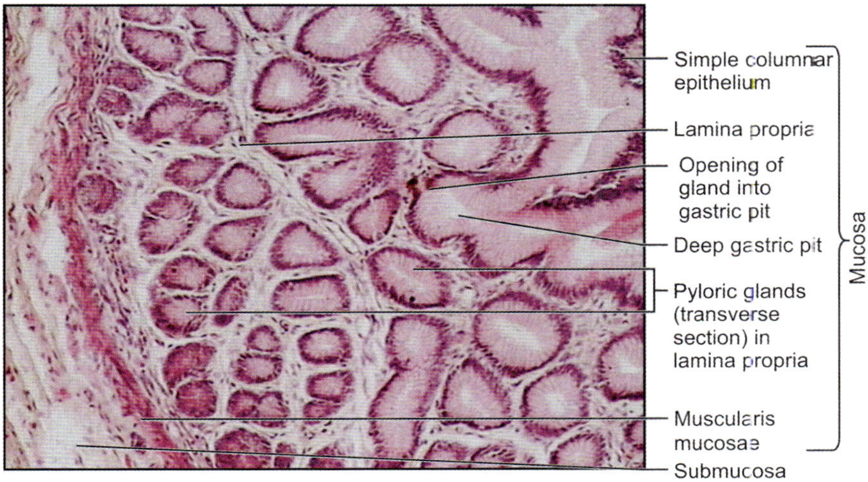

FIGURE 12.13 Stomach pylorus, H & E, X100

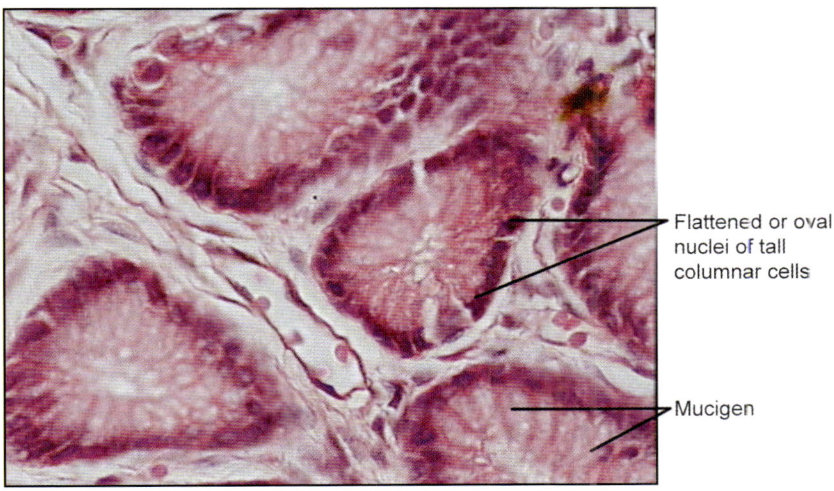

FIGURE 12.14 Stomach pylorus, H & E, X400

The section under high power (Fig. 12.14) shows the pyloric glands. The pyloric glands has mucous cells and enteroendocrine cells intercalated among them. The mucous cells are tall columnar cells that stain lightly due to the mucigen content. The nuclei are flat or oval in shape. The pyloric glands secrete mucous and enzyme lysozyme. The enteroendocrine cells release gastrin and somatostatin.

POINTS TO REMEMBER

Tongue

- Mass of striated muscle covered by mucous membrane.
- Mucous membrane strongly adherent to the muscle.
- Ventral surface of tongue covered by nonkeratinized stratified squamous epithelium.
- Lamina propria thin and closely bound to the underlying muscle.
- Dorsal surface of tongue irregular, covered anteriorly by small eminences called lingual papillae.
  - Posterior 1/3rd contains lymph follicles and lingual tonsils and lined by stratified squamous nonkeratinized epithelium.
  - Anterior 2/3rd contains four types of papillae, which consist of slender vascular core of connective tissue covered by stratified squamous epithelium.
  - Connective tissue core gives rise to small connective tissue papillae, which indent the epithelium.

Filiform papillae	*Fungiform papillae*	*Circumvallate papillae*
• Most numerous and evenly distributed on the anterior 2/3rd of the dorsum of the tongue • Elongated, conical in shape and devoid of taste buds • Lined by stratified squamous keratinized epithelium • Keratin layer tapers into thread-like points	• Relatively few in numbers, interspersed among filiform papillae • Have narrow stalk and smooth surfaced dilated upper part • Lined by stratified squamous nonkeratinized epithelium • Has scattered taste buds	• Seven to twelve in numbers arranged along the V-shaped line • Larger and surrounded by deep groove and wall. • Connective tissue papillae limited to the upper surface. • Circumvallate papillae and the wall covered by stratified squamous nonkeratinized epithelium • Lateral wall of the papillae are the presence of the small oval bodies, the taste buds

Esophagus

Mucosa	Epithelium—stratified squamous nonkeratinized Lamina propria—connective tissue with blood and lymph vessels, lymphatic tissue, glands and smooth muscle cells. Muscularis mucosae—inner circular and outer longitudinal smooth muscle layers
Submucosa	Irregular connective tissue with large blood vessels, lymphatic vessels, Meissner's plexus, esophageal mucous glands and lymphatic tissue in some parts
Muscularis externa	Inner circular and outer longitudinal smooth muscle layers with myenteric (Auerbach's) nerve plexus, blood and lymph vessels - Proximal part, striated muscle; - Middle part both striated and smooth muscle; - Distal part, smooth muscle
Serosa	Loose connective tissue with blood and lymph vessels covered by mesothelium

Stomach

	Fundus	*Pylorus*
Mucosa	Thrown into folds, the rugae	
Epithelium	Simple columnar epithelium continues with the gastric glands	Simple columnar epithelium continues with the gastric glands
Lamina propria	Short gastric pits and long gastric glands Cells lining the glands consist of parietal (oxyntic) cells, chief (zymogenic) cells, mucus neck cells and argentaffin cells.	Long gastric pits and short-coiled tubular pyloric glands. Cells lining the glands consist of mucus secreting and occasionally oxyntic and argentaffin cells
Muscularis mucosa	Inner circular and outer longitudinal	Inner circular and outer longitudinal
Submucosa	Irregular connective tissue with large blood vessels, lymphatic vessels and Meissner's plexus	Irregular connective tissue with large blood vessels, lymphatic vessels and Meissner's plexus
Muscularis externa	Outer longitudinal, middle circular smooth muscle fibers with myenteric (Auerbach's) nerve plexus, blood and lymph vessels and inner oblique smooth muscle layer	Outer longitudinal, middle circular smooth muscle fibers with myenteric (Auerbach's) nerve plexus, blood and lymph vessels and inner oblique smooth muscle layer
Serosa	Loose connective tissue with blood and lymph vessels covered by mesothelium	Loose connective tissue with blood and lymph vessels covered by mesothelium

SMALL INTESTINE

Small intestine, the longest part in the digestive tract is a convoluted tube approximately 5–7 m in length extending from the stomach to the large intestine. The main function of the small intestine is the digestion of gastric contents and absorption of nutrients into the blood capillaries and or lymphatic lacteals.

The small intestine has four layers mucosa, submucosa, muscularis externa and serosa. The mucosa and the submucosa of the small intestine are thrown into permanent spiral folds extending into the lumen, the plicae circulares. Plicae circulares are more prominent in the proximal portion. The lamina propria extends into the intestinal lumen as permanent finger like projections, the villi covered by the simple columnar epithelium. The height of the villi decreases towards the ileum. The connective tissue core of each villus has lymphatic capillary called lacteal, blood capillaries and individual strands of smooth muscle. The lamina propria has intestinal glands or crypts of Lieberkühn located throughout the mucosa. The luminal surfaces of the cells gives the cytoplasmic extensions, the microvilli, which cover the surfaces and give rise to a striated border appearance. Plicae circulares, villi, microvilli increase the absorptive surface area of small intestine. Muscularis mucosae has two layers inner circular and outer longitudinal.

The cells lining the small intestine are columnar absorptive cells, goblet cells, enteroendocrine cells or APUD (amine precursor uptake decarboxylase) cells, mucous cells, undifferentiated cells, Paneth cells, lymphocytes, M (microfold/membrane) cells.

Submucosa has loose connective tissue with blood vessels, lymphatics and nerves.

Muscularis externa has inner circular and outer longitudinal muscle layers.

Serosa is formed by the visceral peritoneum continuous with that of stomach and large intestine. The small intestine is divided into duodenum, jejunum and ileum.

Duodenum

Duodenum is the shortest part of the small intestine. The villi are numerous, broad, tall and look leaf-like. The epithelium is simple columnar and with few goblet cells. Submucosa contains mucus-secreting duodenal glands or Brunner's glands, the characteristic feature of the duodenum.

Section under scanner (Fig. 12.15) shows the mucosa and submucosa. The section shows the finger like projections, the villi towards the luminal surface; the simple columnar cells with microvilli with striated border appearance; the goblet cells stained light and short, tubular intestinal glands in lamina propria. Lamina propria present in the core of the villi has connective tissue cells, lymphoid cells, plasma cells, macrophages, smooth muscle cells, blood vessels and dilated blind ending lymphatic channels, the lacteals. The intestinal glands open into the intervilli spaces. Submucosa shows the mucus secreting cells lining the branched tubuloacinar duodenal glands, the characteristic feature of the duodenum and not present in jejunum, ileum and large intestine. The secretions from the duodenal glands are poured into the base of the intestinal glands through the ducts, which pierce the muscularis mucosae.

Section under low power (Fig. 12.16) shows the mucosa with epithelial layer lined by simple columnar epithelium, intestinal glands in the lamina propria, muscularis mucosae and submucosa. Two types of cells seen in the epithelium are the absorptive cells and goblet cells. Goblet cells are identified by the mucous apical cup, which appears empty in the section. Plicae circulares, villi, microvilli increase the absorptive surface area of small intestine.

Jejunum

Jejunum is the principal site of absorption of nutrients. Jejunum has tall tongue-shaped and few narrow and short finger-like villi and the simple columnar epithelium has more goblet cells.

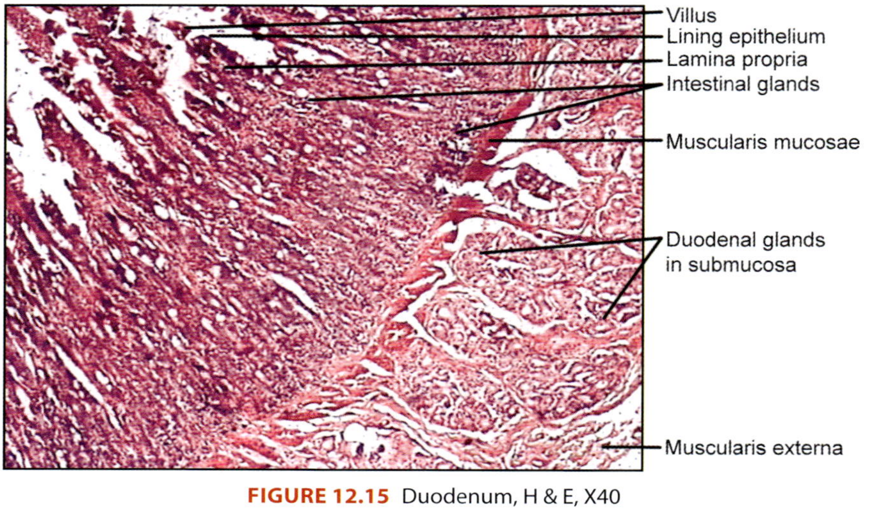

FIGURE 12.15 Duodenum, H & E, X40

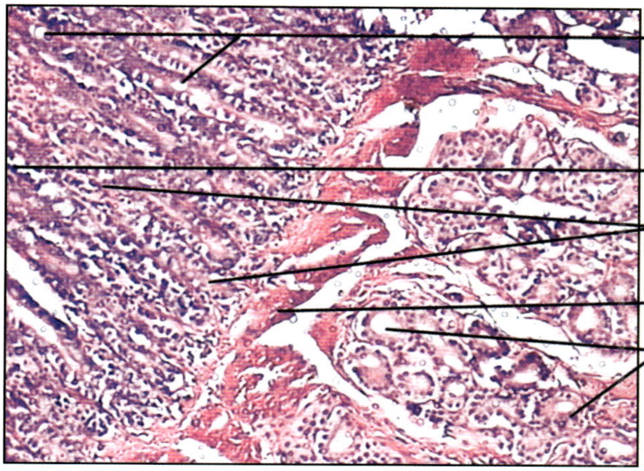

FIGURE 12.16 Duodenum, H & E, X100

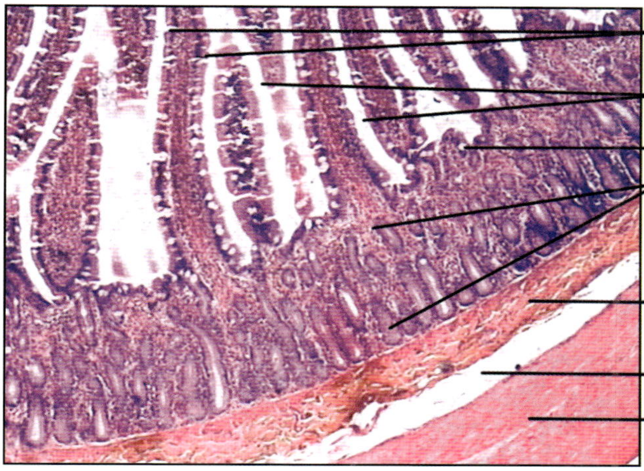

FIGURE 12.17 Jejunum, H & E, X40

Section under scanner (Fig. 12.17) shows the mucosa, submucosa and muscularis externa. The permanent fold of plicae circulares that extend into the lumen and the core of plicae circulares having dense irregular connective tissue submucosa are not seen in this section. The mucosa has epithelial lining, lamina propria with intestinal glands and muscularis mucosae. Villi along with the goblet cells and columnar cells are observed.

Section under the low power (Fig. 12.18) shows the villi with lamina propria in the core of the villi and the mucosa lined by the columnar cells and goblet cells. The villi are epithelial projections into the lumen and the intestinal glands are the epithelial depressions into the wall of the intestine.

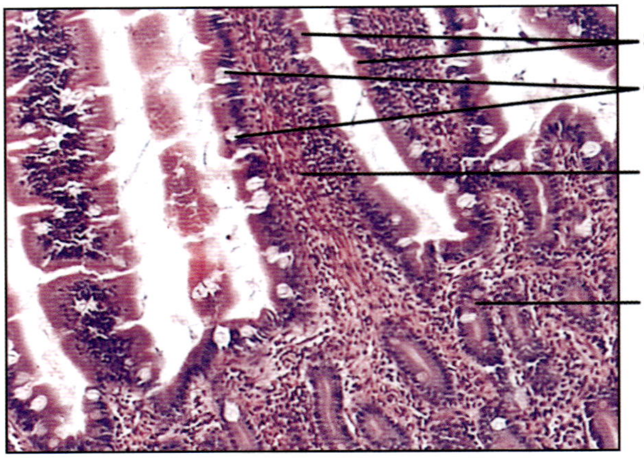

FIGURE 12.18 Jejunum, H & E, X100

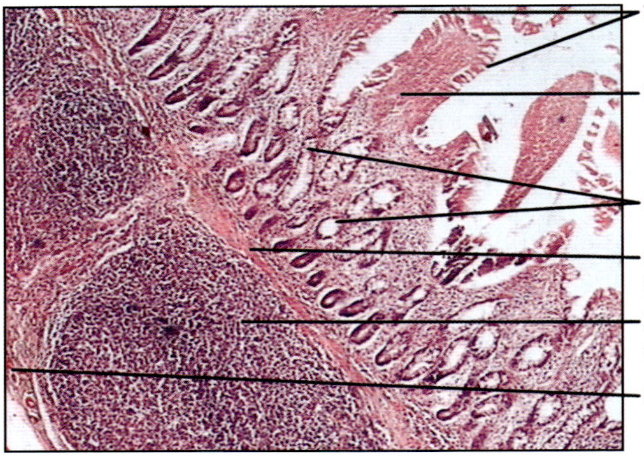

FIGURE 12.19 Ileum, H & E, X40

Ileum

Ileum is the site of water and electrolyte reabsorption. Ileum contains few villi, narrow and short than the jejunum, that look finger-like. The goblet cells in the epithelium are more numerous than duodenum and jejunum. The lymphatic nodules are numerous and large present in the lamina propria and submucosa forming Peyer's patches.

Section under scanner (Fig. 12.19) shows the mucosa and submucosa. The mucosa has the leaf-like villi lined by epithelium with a core of lamina propria. The intestinal glands are present in the lamina propria. The mucosa of the ileum shows distinctive feature, the presence of the single large aggregated lymph nodule forming the Peyer's patch. Sometimes the nodules may extend into the submucosa.

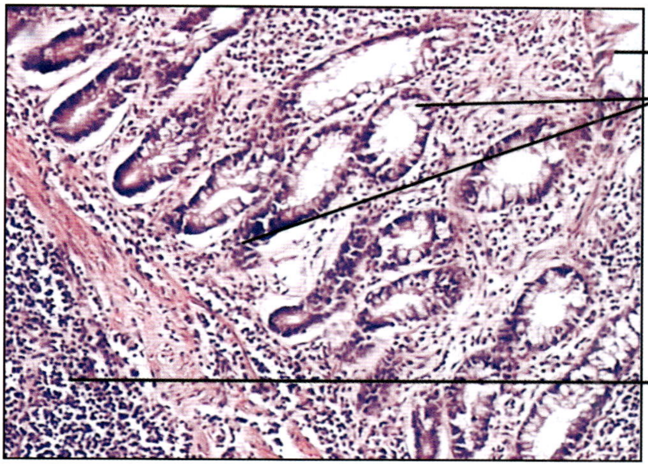

FIGURE 12.20 Ileum, H & E, X100

Section under low power (Fig. 12.20) shows the mucosa. The villi are not appreciated well. Villi should be leaf-like in appearance. A part of the Peyer's patch is seen extending both in mucosa and submucosa and interrupting the muscularis mucosae.

LARGE INTESTINE

Large intestine contains cecum, vermiform appendix, ascending colon, transverse colon, descending colon, rectum and anal canal. The main function of the large intestine is the reabsorption of water and electrolytes especially in the proximal part. The mucus secreted by the goblet cells lubricates the bowel facilitating the passage of solid contents.

The four layers mucosa, submucosa, muscularis externa and serosa are present.

The plicae circulares and villi are absent in the large intestine. Mucosa consists of simple columnar epithelium, intestinal glands, lamina propria and muscularis mucosae. The cells lining the large intestine are mainly columnar absorptive cells and goblet cells. The other cells present are enteroendocrine cells or APUD (amine precursor uptake decarboxylase) cells, mucous cells, undifferentiated cells, lymphocytes, M (microfold/membrane) cells.

The lamina propria has intestinal glands located throughout. Muscularis mucosae consist of two layers inner circular and outer longitudinal.

Submucosa has loose connective tissue with blood vessels, lymphatics and nerves.

Muscularis externa has inner circular and outer longitudinal muscle layers. The arrangement of the outer layer differs from that of small intestine. It is condensed into three prominent longitudinal bands of muscle, called the tenia coli. Between these bands the layer forms a extremely thin sheet. In the rectum, anal canal and vermiform appendix the layer is uniformly thick. The muscularis externa produces segmentation and peristalsis. Segmentation is local and peristalsis results in distal mass movement of colon contents.

Serosa is formed by the visceral peritoneum and on the posterior side it is adventitia.

Sections under scanner (Figs 12.21A and B) shows the four layers, the mucosa, submucosa, muscularis externa and serosa. The plicae circulares and villi are absent. The epithelium is simple

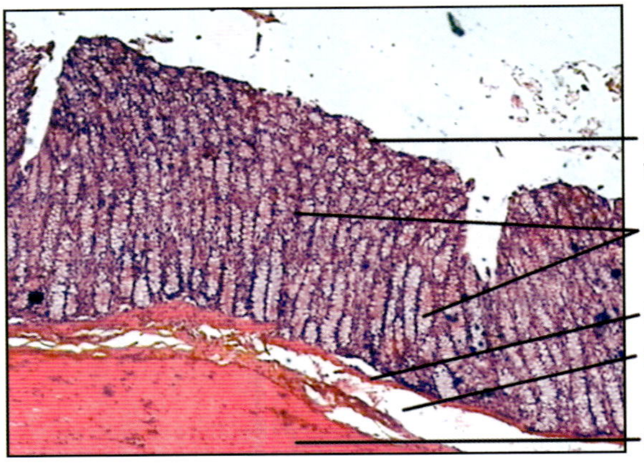

FIGURE 12.21A Large intestine, H & E, X40

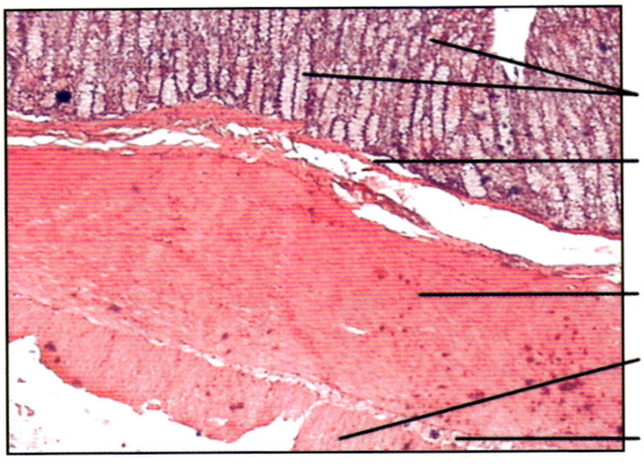

FIGURE 12.21B Large intestine, H & E, X40

columnar epithelium with numerous goblet cells. The lamina propria is filled with intestinal glands. Muscularis mucosae is seen outside to the lamina propria.

Section under low power (Fig. 12.22) shows the intestinal glands with clear numerous goblet cells in the lamina propria. Muscularis mucosae are observed deep to lamina propria.

APPENDIX

Appendix arises from the cecum and intestinal contents may be trapped or sequestered in the appendix, since it is a blind-ended pouch. Plicae circulares and villi are absent, unlike the small intestine.

Section under scanner (Fig. 12.23) shows the mucosa, submucosa and muscularis externa. The lamina propria shows the intestinal glands, diffuse lymphatic tissue and lymph nodules. The lamina propria and submucosa blends with each other. The deeper part of the submucosa has blood vessels

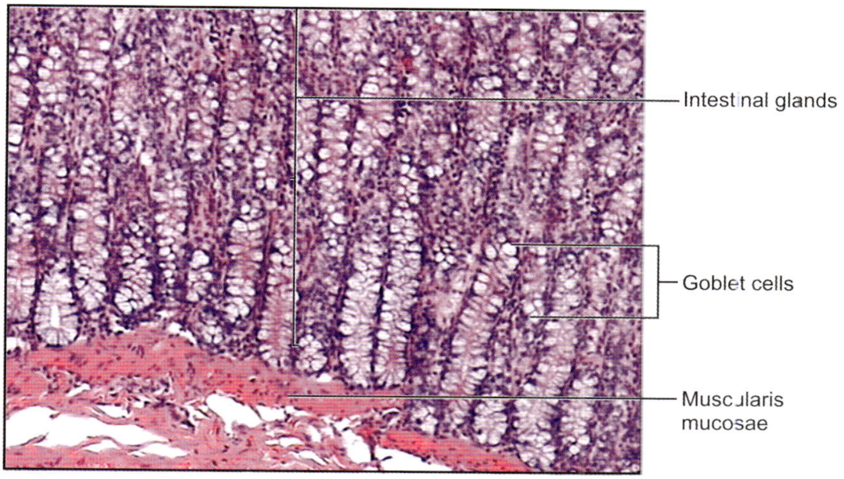

FIGURE 12.22 Large intestine, H & E, X100

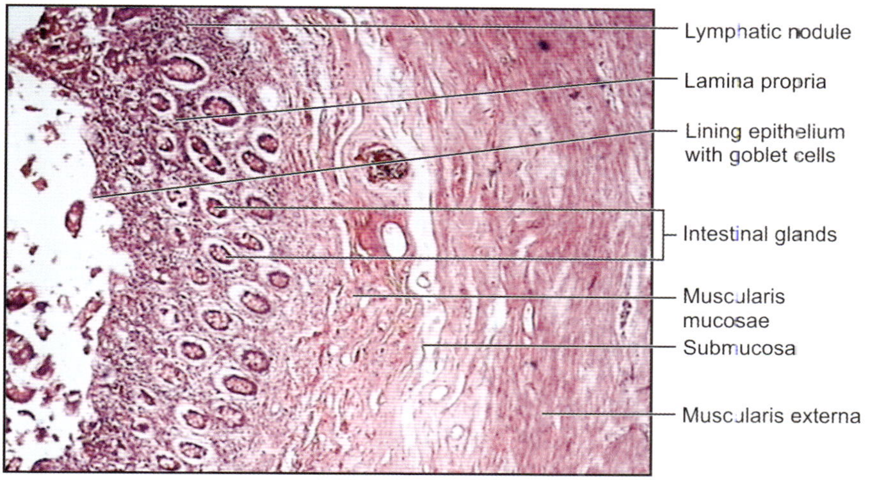

FIGURE 12.23 Appendix, H & E, X40

and nerves. Muscularis externa has inner thick circular muscle and outer thin longitudinal muscle layer.

Section under low power (Fig. 12.24) shows the intestinal glands, disrupted muscularis mucosae not very well-appreciated and submucosa. The epithelium shows numerous light stained goblet cells, Paneth cells and argentaffin cells. The lamina propria is heavily infiltrated with lymphocytes with disrupted muscularis mucosae.

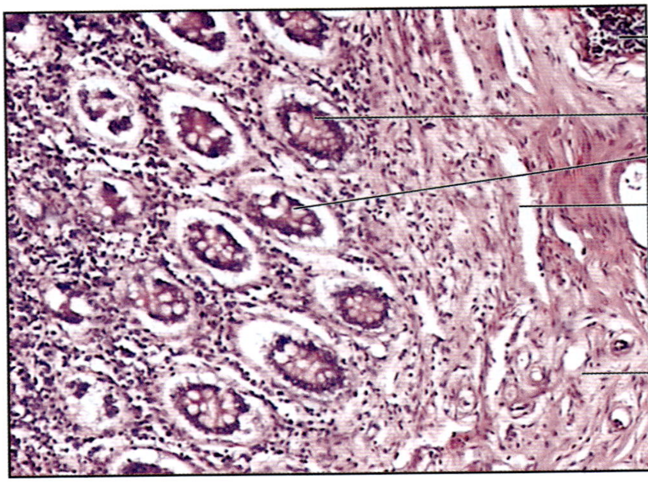

FIGURE 12.24 Appendix, H & E, X100

POINTS TO REMEMBER

Duodenum, Jejunum, Ileum

	Duodenum	*Jejunum*	*Ileum*
Mucosa			
• Epithelium	Striated columnar with few goblets cells	Striated columnar with more goblet cells	Striated columnar with a high number of goblet cells
• Villi	Leaf-shaped crypts with argentaffin cells	Tall, tongue-shaped crypts with less argentaffin cells	Short, finger-shaped crypts with less argentaffin cells
• Lamina propria	Loose lymphatic tissue.	Diffuse lymphatic nodules	Lymphatic nodules aggregated to form Peyer's patches
Muscularis mucosa	Continuous	Interrupted	Interrupted
Submucosa	Presence of Brunner's glands. Connective tissue with blood vessels and nerves	Connective tissue with blood vessels and nerves	Presence of Peyer's patches. Connective tissue with blood vessels and nerves
Muscularis externa	Inner circular and outer longitudinal smooth muscle layers with myenteric (Auerbach's) nerve plexus, blood and lymph vessels	Inner circular and outer longitudinal smooth muscle layers with myenteric (Auerbach's) nerve plexus, blood and lymph vessels	Inner circular and outer longitudinal smooth muscle layers with myenteric (Auerbach's) nerve plexus, blood and lymph vessels
Serosa	Loose connective tissue with blood and lymph vessels covered by mesothelium	Loose connective tissue with blood and lymph vessels covered by mesothelium	Loose connective tissue with blood and lymph vessels covered by mesothelium

Appendix

Mucosa Epithelium	Many goblet cells, some Paneth cells and a number of argentaffin cells
Lamina propria	Connective tissue with blood and lymph vessels, lymphatic tissue. Occupied by a continuous ring of lymphoid nodules, which invade submucosa through muscularis mucosae. Difficult to separate lamina propria and submucosa. Taenia coli absent.
Muscularis mucosae	Inner circular and outer longitudinal smooth muscle layers.
Submucosa	Irregular connective tissue with large blood vessels, lymphatic vessels, Meissner's plexus, lymphatic nodules.
Muscularis externa	Inner circular and outer longitudinal smooth muscle layers with myenteric (Auerbach's) nerve plexus, blood and lymph vessels.
Serosa	Loose connective tissue with blood and lymph vessels, covered by mesothelium.

Small Intestine and Large Intestine

	Small intestine	*Large intestine*
Mucosa	Plicae circulares and villi present	Absent
Epithelium	Goblet cells less in number and columnar cells more in number	Goblet cells more in number and few columnar cells
Lamina propria	Crypts of Lieberkühn are few and consist of columnar cells, goblet cells, more number of Paneth and argentaffin cells	Crypts are more numerous, deeper and consists of less number of columnar cells,numerous goblet cells, very rarely Paneth and argentaffin cells
Muscularis mucosa	Smooth muscle: Inner circular and outer longitudinal layers. Interrupted in some regions	Smooth muscle: Inner circular and outer longitudinal layers
Submucosa	Irregular connective tissue with large blood vessels, lymphatic vessels, Meissner's plexus, glands and lymphatic tissue in some parts	Irregular connective tissue with large blood vessels, lymphatic vessels, Meissner's plexus, lymphatic tissue
Muscularis externa	Inner circular and outer longitudinal smooth muscle layers with myenteric (Auerbach's) nerve plexus, blood and lymph vessels. Longitudinal coat uniformly thick	Inner circular and outer longitudinal smooth muscle layers with myenteric (Auerbach's) nerve plexus, blood and lymph vessels. Longitudinal coat, thickened to form three bands, the taenia coli
Serosa	Loose connective tissue covered by mesothelium, has blood and lymph vessels	In some parts absent, which are covered by adventitia

Cells in Gastrointestinal Tract

	Parietal cells	*Chief cells*	*Argentaffin cells*	*Goblet cells*	*Paneth cells*
Location	Mostly in the upper half of gastric glands, along with mucous neck cells	Mostly in the lower region of gastric glands	At the base of the glands, along with chief cells	Lining epithelium, more towards large intestine	Base of intestinal glands in the small intestine
Cells	Rounded or pyramidal cells, central spherical nuclei, eosinophilic cytoplasm	Pyramidal cells, basophilic granular cytoplasm	Dense secretory granules at the base, have high affinity for silver or chromium salts, because of which, the nuclei are not properly visible	Pear-shaped cells	Serozymogenic cells with chromophilic material at the base and acidophilic secretory granules at the apex
Secretion	Hydrochloric acid	Pepsin	Serotonin	Mucus. At the points of discharge of secretion, surface membrane not modified. As the secretion increases, mucus displaces the cytoplasm and nucleus is flattened	Digestive enzymes

LIVER

Liver is the largest glandular tissue in the body. Liver produces and secretes many circulating plasma proteins. Liver plays an important role in the uptake, storage and distribution of nutrients and vitamins from bloodstream. It maintains the blood glucose level, regulates circulating levels of very low density lipoproteins, degrades or conjugates numerous toxic substances and drugs, produces bile secretion containing bile salts, phospholipids and cholesterol. Absorbed food products and liquids from the digestive organs first percolate through liver capillaries, called the sinusoids. Nutrient-rich blood in the hepatic portal vein is brought to the liver before it enters the general circulation. Because venous blood from the digestive organs is poor in oxygen, the hepatic artery from the aorta supplies liver cells with oxygenated blood supply to the liver. Liver has exocrine and endocrine functions.

The structure of the liver is described in three ways in terms of functional unit, the classic lobule, the portal lobule and liver acinus. The liver has hexagonal units the classic or liver or hepatic lobules. From the central vein present in the center of each lobule, plates of liver cells, the hepatocytes and the sinusoids radiate towards the periphery. Here connective tissue forms portal triads containing the branches of hepatic artery, hepatic portal vein and bile duct. Venous and arterial blood first mix in liver sinusoids as they flow toward the central vein. Between portal triad and hepatic laminae is the space of Mall. From the space of Mall, blood enters the general circulation through the hepatic veins that leave the liver. The portal lobule is triangular in shape and the outer margins are imaginary lines drawn between the three central veins that are closest to portal triad. These lines define a roughly triangular block of tissue that includes those portions of three classic lobules that secrete bile that drains into its axial bile duct. The liver acinus is lozenge or diamond-shaped in structure. The short axis is defined by the terminal branches of portal triad that lies along the border between two classic lobules. The long axis is a line drawn between the two central veins closest to short axis occupying two parts of adjacent classic lobules.

Hepatic sinusoids are tortuous, dilated blood channels lined by a discontinuous layer of fenestrated endothelial cells. The endothelial cells are separated from the underlying hepatocytes by the perisinusoidal space of Disse. As a result ingested material carried in the sinusoids enters the discontinuous endothelial wall and comes in direct contact with hepatocytes. The structure and path of the sinusoids through the liver allows an efficient exchange of materials between the hepatocytes and blood. Sinusoids are not only lined by the endothelial cells but also by the phagocytic Kupffer cells, which can be demonstrated by intravenous injection of India ink.

Hepatocytes secrete bile into tiny channels, called the bile canaliculi that are located between the individual hepatocytes. The canaliculi converge at the periphery of each liver lobule in the portal areas as bile ducts. The bile ducts then drain into larger hepatic ducts that carry bile out of the liver. Within the liver lobules, bile flows in bile canaliculi toward the bile duct in the portal triad whereas blood in the sinusoids flows toward the central vein, hence bile and blood do not mix. The hepatocytes filled with glycogen granules after the meals can be demonstrated by periodic acid-Schiff staining. Reticular fibers provide most of the supporting connective tissue of the liver; line the sinusoids, support the endothelial cells and form dense network of reticular fibers in the wall of central vein. Reticular fibers can be demonstrated by the silver impregnation technique.

Section under scanner (Fig. 12.25) shows the hepatic lobules with central vein, hepatocytes, sinusoids and portal triad. Central vein is present in the center of the lobule from which the plates of

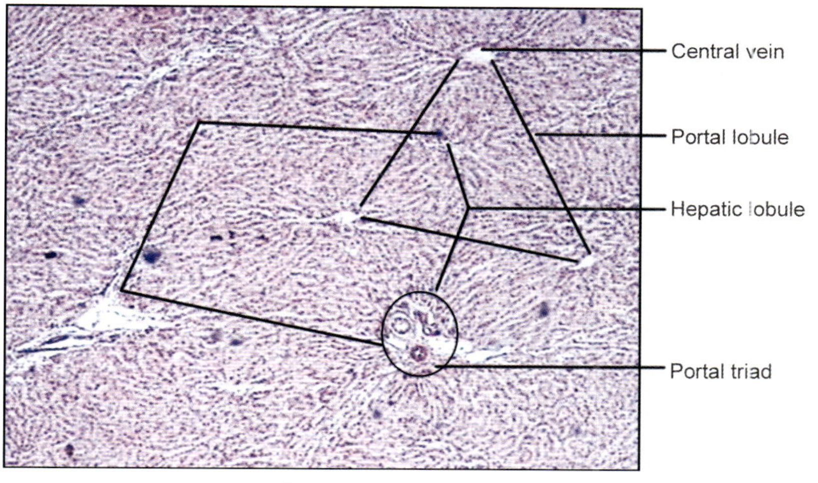

FIGURE 12.25 Liver, H & E, X40

hepatocytes radiate towards the periphery. Portal triad contains the interlobular branches of portal vein, bile duct and hepatic artery. The connective tissue septa between the hepatic lobules are not distinctly made out. The portal lobule identified in this section is between the three central veins.

Section under low power (Fig. 12.26) shows one incomplete hepatic lobule with central vein, hepatocytes, sinusoids and portal triad. Hepatic sinusoids are present between the hepatic plates which appear as clear spaces between the hepatic plates. The hepatic cells appear as one or more cell thick interconnecting cords, but are arranged in one cell thick plates. The nuclei of hepatocytes are clearly visible.

Section under high power (Fig. 12.27) shows central vein with hepatocytes and sinusoids. The continuation of the sinusoids with the central vein is seen. The polygonal shape, nuclei and nucleoli of the hepatocytes and nuclei of the sinusoidal endothelium can be identified. The endothelium can be identified by the flat appearance of the nuclei. In some hepatocyte cells, lipid droplets are

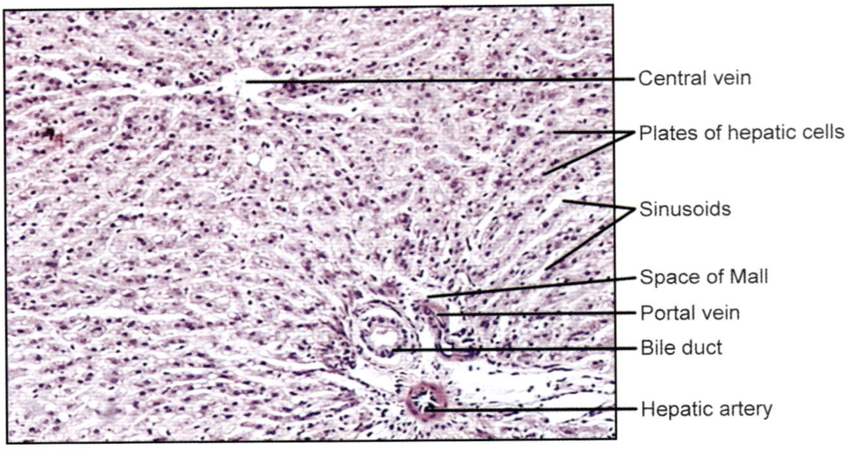

FIGURE 12.26 Liver, H & E, X100

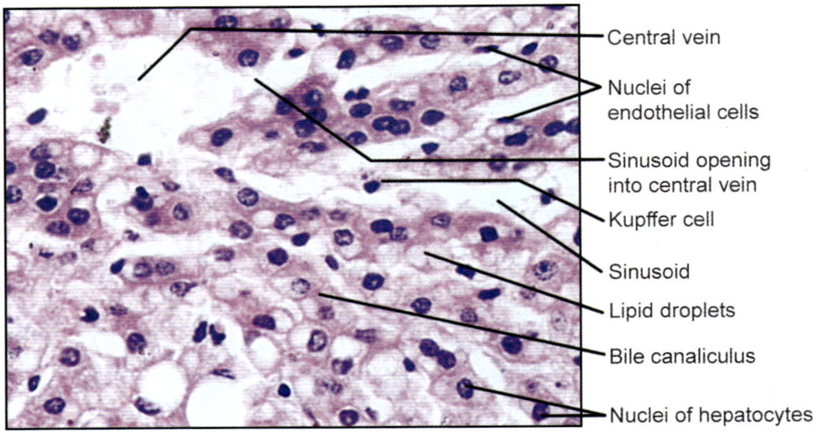

FIGURE 12.27 Liver, H & E, X400

present. Apart from endothelial cells Kupffer cells, phagocytic in nature lining the sinusoid can be identified. Kupffer cells have large nucleus and protrude into the lumen. Bile canaliculi between two hepatocytes are clearly visible.

GALLBLADDER

The gallbladder is a pear-shaped small hollow muscular organ attached to the inferior surface of the liver. Bile produced by liver hepatocytes flows to and is stored in the gallbladder. Bile leaves the gallbladder via the cystic duct and enters the duodenum via the common bile duct through the major duodenal papilla, a finger-like protrusion of the duodenal wall into the lumen. Gallbladder is not a gland and the function is to store and concentrate bile which is released into the digestive tract as a result of hormonal stimulation after a meal. Mucosa of gallbladder shows deep folds in the empty state.

Section under scanner (Fig. 12.28) shows the mucosa, muscularis and adventitia or serosa. Simple columnar epithelium and underlying connective tissue, lamina propria are observed in the mucosa. The temporary mucosal folds varying in size and shape observed when the gallbladder is empty and the folds disappear, once it is filled with bile.

Cross-section of the invaginated epithelium into the lamina propria as well as into the muscular layer is called Rokitansky-Aschoff sinus.

Muscular layer has randomly arranged smooth muscle fibers. There is no distinct arrangement of the fibers. Adventitia consists of thick layer of dense connective tissue with large blood vessels, lymphatics and nerves, which forms adventitia towards the attached surface and the unattached surface is covered by the peritoneum forming the serosa.

Section under low power (Fig. 12.29) shows the mucosa and muscular layers. Tall simple columnar epithelium absorptive in nature and diverticulum or crypt is seen in the mucosal layer. Blood vessel is seen in the lamina propria that is usually cellular. Randomly arranged smooth muscles are identified.

PANCREAS

Pancreas soft elongated organ is located posterior to the stomach. Pancreas contains separate exocrine and endocrine parts.

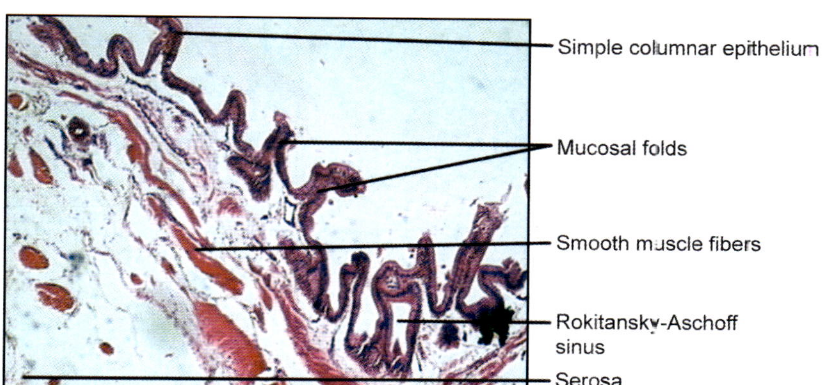

FIGURE 12.28 Gallbladder, H & E, X40

Exocrine part forms most of the pancreas. The exocrine part is a compound tubuloacinar gland having secretory units or acini with pyramid-shaped acinar cells, the apices of which filled with secretory granules containing the precursors of the several pancreatic inactive digestive enzymes. The acini are divided into lobules by loose connective tissue. The excretory ducts start from within the center of the individual acini as pale staining centroacinar cells that continue into the short intercalated ducts. Intercalated ducts merge to form intralobular ducts in the connective tissue and these ducts join to form larger interlobular ducts emptying into the main pancreatic duct.

Endocrine part is scattered among the exocrine acini as isolated units and the pale staining vascularized units are the pancreatic islets of Langerhans. Each islet is surrounded by fine fibers of reticular connective tissue. There are four types of cells, the alpha (A/α 15–20%), beta (B/β 70%), delta (D/δ 5-10%) and pancreatic polypeptide cells (F/PP) (5%).

Section under scanner (Fig. 12.30) shows both darkly stained exocrine and lightly stained endocrine parts. The exocrine part forms most of the pancreas and consists of closely packed serous

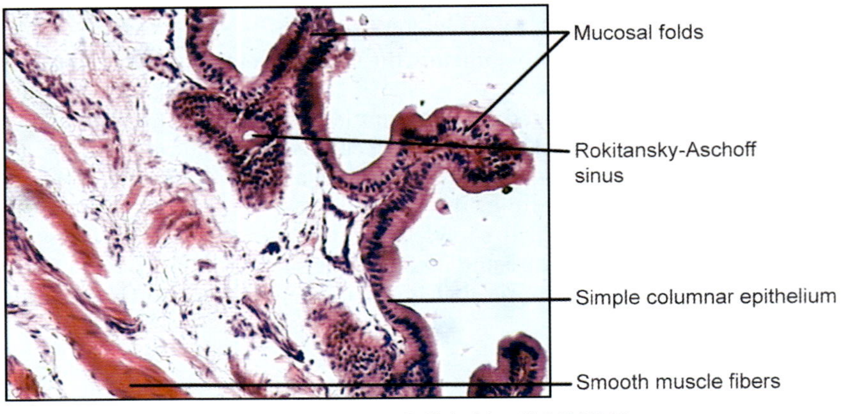

FIGURE 12.29 Gallbladder, H & E, X100

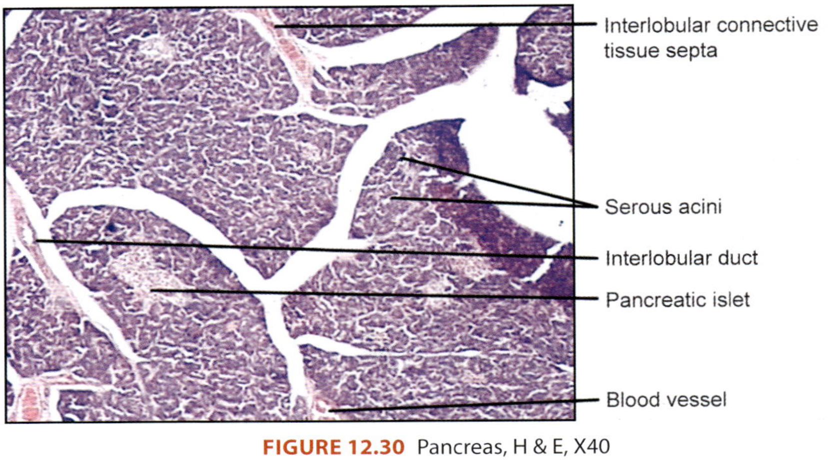

FIGURE 12.30 Pancreas, H & E, X40

acini and zymogenic cells arranged into small lobules. The acini are surrounded by intralobular connective tissue and the lobules by interlobular connective tissue. Interlobular connective tissue contains blood vessels and interlobular duct. The white empty spaces between the lobules are artifacts, may be because the connective tissue is washed off during the preparation.

Section under low power (Fig. 12.31) shows the lobules with the exocrine and endocrine parts. Each pancreatic acinus consists of pyramid-shaped protein secreting zymogenic cells that surround irregular central lumen, which appears as white spaces. The centroacinar cells are seen within the lumina as pale staining cells. The cells in pancreatic islets are arranged in cords and clumps. Between the cords are the connective tissue fibers and capillary network.

Section under high power (Fig. 12.32) shows the different types of cells in the pancreatic islet. The cytoplasm of the alpha cells stain pink and cells are situated more peripherally in the islet and secrete glucagons. The cytoplasm of beta cells stain blue and beta cells are situated in the center.

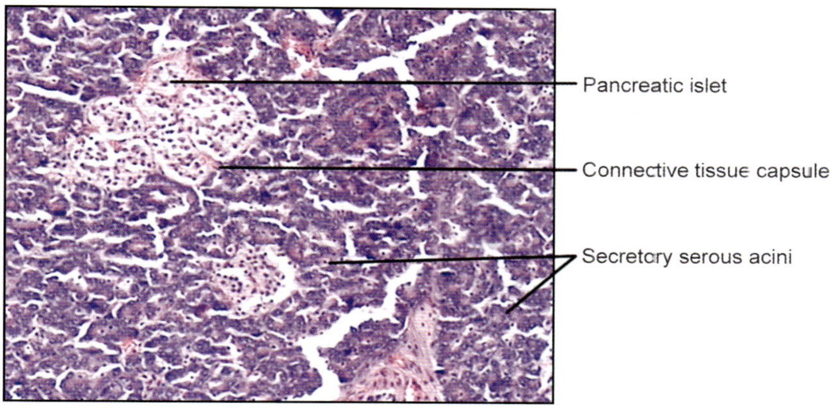

FIGURE 12.31 Pancreas, H & E, X100

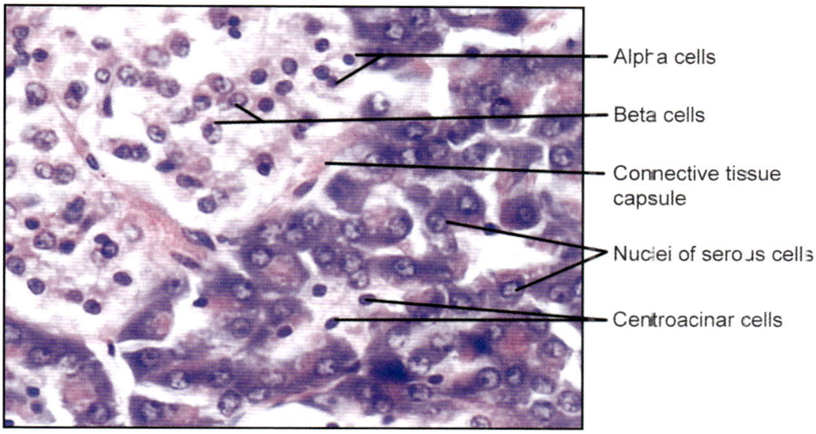

FIGURE 12.32 Pancreas, H & E, X400

Capillaries identified demonstrate rich vascularity. The islets and the serous acini are separated by thin connective tissue capsule.

POINTS TO REMEMBER

Liver

- Largest gland of the body. Covered by Glisson's capsule, which at porta hepatis surrounds the blood vessels and divides the gland into small innumerable hepatic lobules.
- *Hepatic lobule:* Hepatic cells in the order of hepatic laminae radiate from the central vein to the periphery limited by six portal triads containing branches of hepatic artery, portal vein and interlobular bile ductule and interlobular connective tissue.
- *Space of Mall:* Potential space between the portal triad and hepatic laminae.
- Lobules are continuous with each other in human. Spaces between the hepatic laminae are the hepatic sinusoids, lined by reticular endothelial cells and Kupffer (phagocytic) cells.
- *Space of Disse:* Space between the sinusoids and hepatic laminae.
- Two surfaces of hepatic cell are related to the sinusoids and the other four surfaces to the bile canaliculi.
- *Functions:* Secretion (bile), storage (fat, protein, vitamins, carbohydrate) and excretion (removal of waste products from blood).
- *Views:* Histological architecture of liver:
  - Hepatic lobule
  - Portal lobule
  - Portal acinus.

Gallbladder

Mucosa	Thrown into temporary folds.
• Epithelium	Simple tall columnar epithelium with brush border. Cross-section of the invaginated epithelium into the lamina propria as well as into the muscular layer is called Rokitansky-Aschoff sinus.
• Lamina Propria	Loose connective tissue with diffused lymphatic tissue. Glands absent.
Fibromuscular layer	Smooth muscle interspersed with loose connective tissue rich in elastic fibers.
Perimuscular layer	Loose connective tissue with blood vessels, lymphatics and nerves.
Serosa/adventitia	Mesothelium covering loose connective tissue. Serosa on its free surface/ adventitia on attached surface.
Function	Acts as reservoir for bile production.

Pancreas

- Pancreas has both exocrine and endocrine parts.
- Loose connective tissue divides it into small lobules.

Exocrine Part

- Serous acini lined by irregular pyramidal cells.
- Cells have zymogen granules towards the apex and chromophilic substance towards the base. Nuclei lie towards the basal zone.
- Acini continuous with the intercalated ducts (intralobular), which join together to form interlobular ducts,leading to the main excretory duct.
- Striated ducts absent.
- Secretes pancreatic juice consisting of trypsin, amylase and lipase.

Endocrine Part (Islets of Langerhans)

- Present irregularly among the acini or along the ducts.
- Arranged as irregular anastomosing cords.
- Between the cells are numerous blood capillaries.
- Only few fine connective tissue fibers are present.
- Three types of cells: α or alpha cells, B or beta cells and D cells.
- Also present are the F/PP cells.

α, β, δ and F/PP Cells

	A/α (alpha) cells	B/β (beta) cells	D/δ (delta)/ Type III cells	F/PP cells
Cells	Numerous, fine, red staining granules and distinct cell membrane	More numerous than alpha cells with dark blue coarse granules and indistinct cell membrane	Placed peripherally, stain with silver salts	Mostly present in head and neck of pancreas
Secretion	Glucagons	Insulin and amylin	Somatostatin	Pancreatic polypeptide

CHAPTER 13

Urinary System

Urinary system consists of two kidneys, two ureters, single urinary bladder and single urethra.

KIDNEY

The freshly cut kidney has two parts, the outer cortex and the inner medulla, which consist of numerous renal pyramids. The kidney is covered by connective tissue capsule. The base of each renal pyramid faces the cortex and the apex form the renal papilla in the renal pelvis. A part of the cortex extends on either side of the renal pyramids to form the renal columns. Each renal papilla is surrounded by funnel-shaped minor calyx, which in turn joins to form the major calyx. The major calyces join to form the renal pelvis that leaves the hilum of the kidney and becomes continuous with the ureter.

The functional and structural unit of kidney is nephron. There are about 2 million nephrons in each human kidney. Nephrons are responsible for the production of urine. The nephron is made up of the renal corpuscle and the renal tubule. The renal corpuscle consists of the glomerulus, a tuft of capillary loops that is surrounded by a double-layered epithelial cup, the renal or Bowman's capsule. The glomerular capillaries are supplied at the vascular pole of Bowman's capsule by an afferent arteriole and drained by an efferent arteriole that leaves Bowman's capsule at the vascular pole and then branches to form a new capillary network to supply the kidney tubules. Opposite to the vascular pole is the urinary pole, where the filtrate leaves the renal capsule. The tubular parts of the nephron are arranged in three segments—the proximal thick segment (proximal convoluted tubule and the proximal straight tubule), the thin segment (constitutes the thin limb of the loop of Henle), and the distal thick segment (distal straight tubule and the distal convoluted tubule). The thick straight portions of the proximal and distal tubules are the thick segment of the loop of Henle and the thin segment between them form the U-shaped loop of Henle. The distal convoluted tubule joins the collecting tubule. The nephron and the collecting tubule together form the uriniferous tubule.

The cortex contains the renal corpuscles, numerous proximal convoluted tubules and few distal convoluted tubules. The medullary ray in the cortex has straight descending segment of proximal convoluted tubules, straight ascending segments of the distal convoluted tubules and the collecting tubules. The medulla contains straight portions of the tubules and parts of loop of Henle (thick and thin descending segments, thin and thick ascending segments).

Section under scanner (Fig. 13.1) shows the renal cortex divided into cortical labyrinth and medullary rays. The cortical labyrinth contains the renal corpuscles. Surrounding each renal corpuscle are the proximal and distal convoluted tubules. The medullary rays are composed of groups of straight tubules oriented in the same direction and appear to radiate from the base of the pyramid. The medullary rays are cut longitudinally; hence the tubules present elongated profiles. The medullary rays contain proximal straight tubules (thick segment of the descending limb of loop of Henle) distal straight tubules (thick segment of the ascending limb of loop of Henle) and collecting tubules.

Section under low power (Fig. 13.2) shows the cortex with the renal corpuscle and the tubules (round and oval). The proximal convoluted tubules are lined by cuboidal cells having brush border

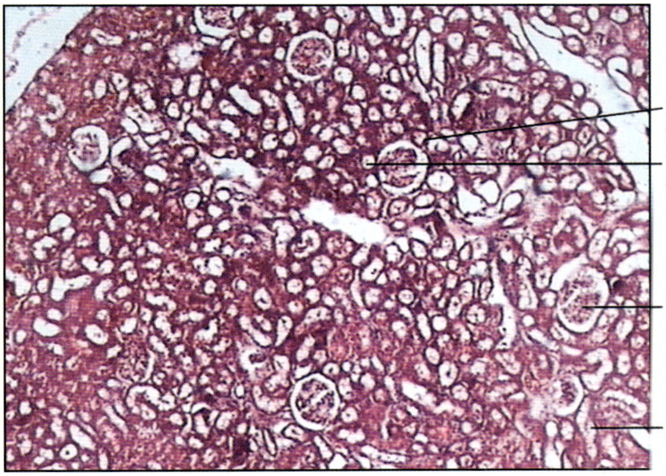

FIGURE 13.1 Kidney, H & E, X40

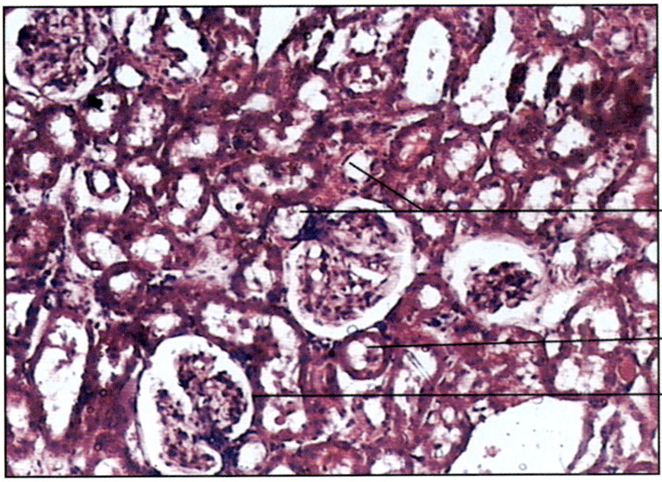

FIGURE 13.2 Kidney, H & E, X100

and have an uneven star-shaped lumen; but the distal convoluted tubules have, larger lumen with smaller cuboidal cells. Typically, fewer nuclei appear in a cross-section of proximal tubule than in the distal tubule. The number of proximal and distal convoluted tubules is equal in the medullary ray, but the distal convoluted tubules are less in the cortex.

Section under high power (Fig. 13.3) shows the renal corpuscle with juxtaglomerular apparatus. The periphery is composed of a thin capsule, the Bowman's capsule enclosing a narrow clear space, the urinary space and a capillary tuft or glomerulus. The capsule has two parts: Parietal layer and visceral layer. The parietal layer consists of simple squamous epithelial cells. The visceral layer consists of podocytes that lie on the outer surface of the glomerular capillary. Podocytes may be difficult to distinguish from the capillary endothelial cells. Nuclei of podocytes are larger and stain less intensely than the nuclei of the endothelial and mesangial cells.

The cells of the distal convoluted tubule adjacent to the afferent arteriole are narrow, columnar and more crowded on one side constituting the macula densa. The vascular pole is characterized by the presence of arterioles one of which enter or leave the corpuscle. The afferent arteriole possesses modified smooth muscle cells with granules, the juxtaglomerular cells. Adjacent to the glomerulus are the mesangial cells. The macula densa, juxtaglomerular cells and mesangial cells together form the juxtaglomerular apparatus. At the urinary pole, the parietal layer of the Bowman's capsule becomes continuous with the lumen of the proximal convoluted tubule and the lining cells change from simple squamous to simple cuboidal or low columnar with brush border.

URETER

The ureters are paired tubular structures that convey urine from the kidneys to the urinary bladder. The wall consists of mucosa, muscularis and adventitia. In the empty state, the lumen is irregular and star-shaped. Mucosa is lined by the transitional epithelium. Urine passes in the ureter then the wall distends, since the epithelium becomes thinner and flatter. Lamina propria contains dense fibroelastic connective tissue with more fibroblasts; diffuse lymphatic tissue and occasional small lymphatic nodules. Muscularis consists of inner longitudinal and outer circular smooth muscle layers that are not distinct in the upper part of the ureter and in the lower third there is an additional

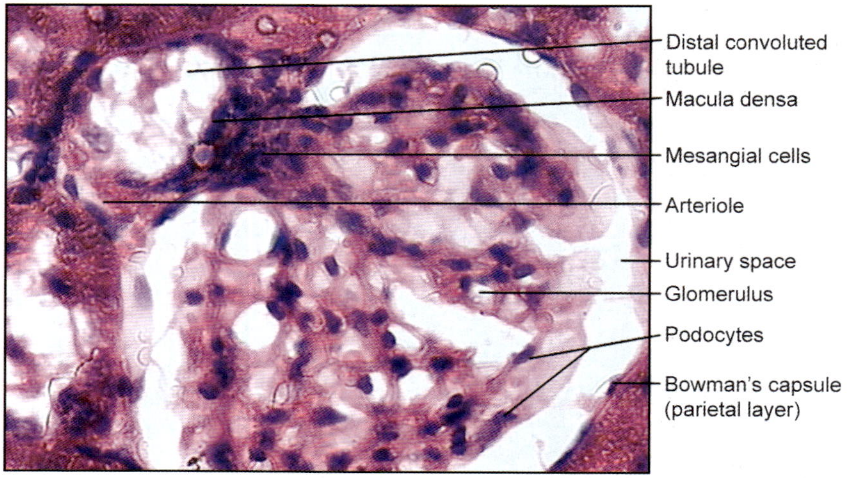

FIGURE 13.3 Kidney, H & E, X400

outer longitudinal smooth muscle layer. Regular peristaltic contractions of the muscle contribute to the flow of urine from the kidney to the urinary bladder. Adventitia blends with the surrounding connective tissue and adipose tissue and has the arterioles, venules and small nerves.

Section under scanner (Fig. 13.4) shows the three layers of ureter, the mucosa, muscularis and adventitia. The highly folded mucosa is lined by the transitional epithelium. The transitional epithelium has several layers. The lamina propria has fibroelastic connective tissue with fibroblasts and diffuse lymphatic tissue. A distinct submucosa is not present, although the term is sometimes applied to the connective tissue that is closest to the muscle. The three layers of muscularis are arranged as an inner longitudinal layer, a middle circular layer and an outer longitudinal layer.

Section under low power (Fig. 13.5) shows the transitional epithelium, lamina propria and inner longitudinal smooth muscle layer. The transitional epithelium shows the basal cells being the

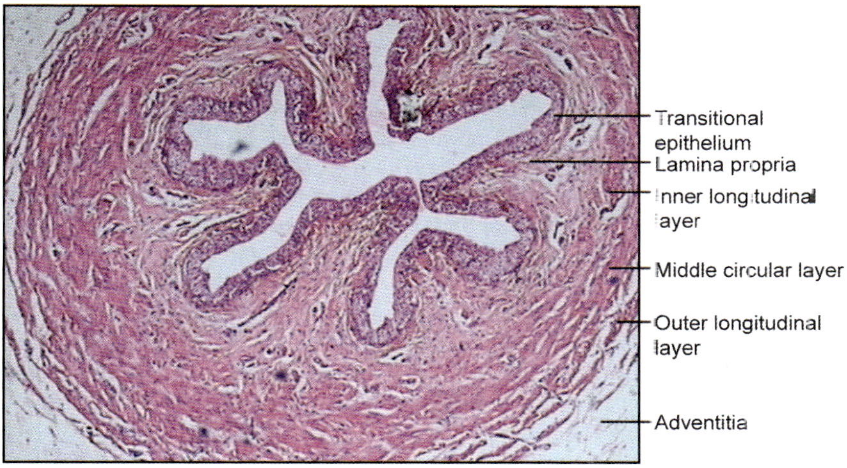

FIGURE 13.4 Ureter, H & E, X40

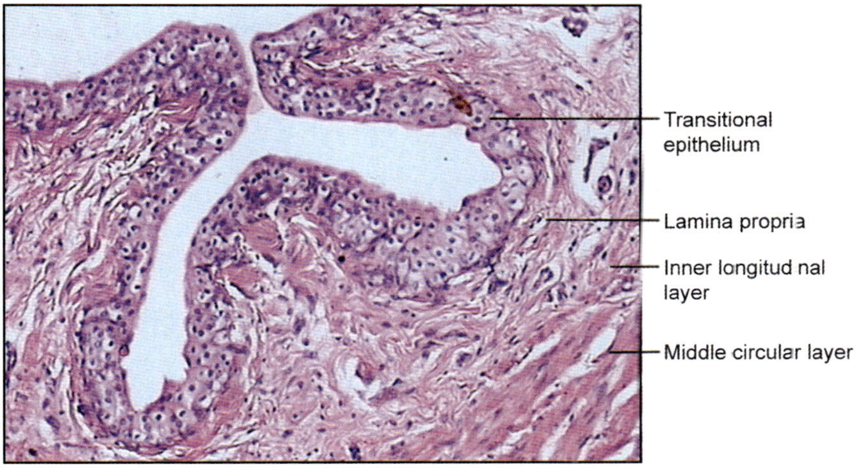

FIGURE 13.5 Ureter, H & E, X100

low columnar or cuboidal, middle cells polyhedral and surface cells large cuboidal. The basal cells are the smallest with the nuclei appearing crowded, because of the minimal cytoplasm of each cell. The intermediate cells are larger in size than the basal cells, but smaller than the surface cells. The epithelium and the lamina propria are separated by a thin basement membrane. In the muscularis, the nuclei appear as round profiles, indicating that the muscle cells are cut transversely.

URINARY BLADDER

The urinary bladder receives the urine from the two ureters and stores it until neural stimulation causes it to contract and expel the urine via the urethra. The urinary bladder consists of mucosa, muscularis and serosa on the superior surface and adventitia on the inferior surface. The mucosa is thrown into numerous folds when bladder is empty and is lined by the transitional epithelium. The lamina propria is wider than in the ureter and consists of more elastic fibers. The muscularis is very thick and has three layers that are not distinguishable from each other. They are arranged in anastomosing bundles with interstitial connective tissue and blood vessels. The interstitial connective tissue merges with the serosa.

Section under scanner (Fig. 13.6) shows mucosa and muscularis. Numerous mucosal folds are observed that are lined by the transitional epithelium. Beneath the epithelium is a relatively thick layer of lamina propria containing connective tissue and blood vessels of various sizes. The muscularis consists of smooth muscles arranged in three indistinct layers. As the ureter passes through the bladder wall, it carries a layer of longitudinally oriented smooth muscle along with it. Medium-sized arteries and veins are occasionally seen in the muscularis.

Section under low power (Fig. 13.7) shows the transitional epithelium and the underlying connective tissue. The surface cells of transitional epithelium are low cuboidal or columnar, which appear dome-shaped. Some of the cells may be binucleate. The outer plasma membrane is thickened in the superficial cells called plaques, which help cells to expand, during distention. The thickness of the transitional epithelium is variable. When the bladder stretches, the superficial cells become squamous and as few as three layers are seen and in the contracted bladder, it appears as though as many as ten layers are present. The lamina propria contains fine connective tissue fibers,

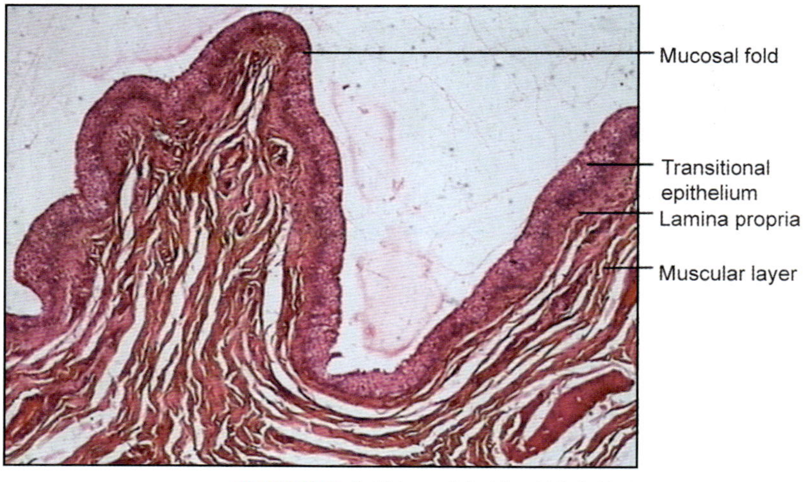

FIGURE 13.6 Urinary bladder, H & E, X40

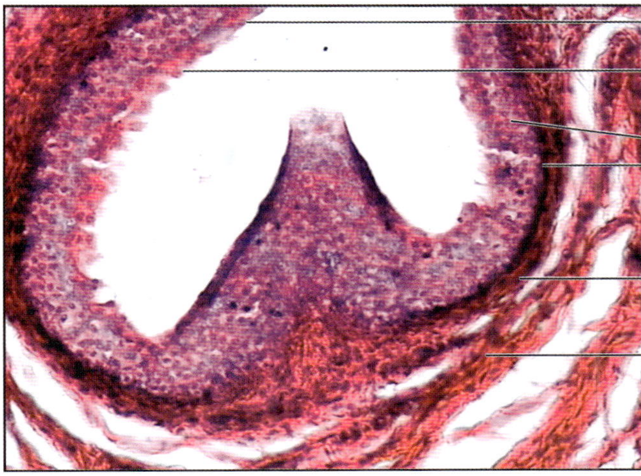

FIGURE 13.7 Urinary bladder, H & E, X100

numerous fibroblasts and blood vessels. Adjacent to the mucosa are bundles of longitudinally sectioned smooth muscle.

POINTS TO REMEMBER

Kidney

Nephron is the functional and the structural unit of kidney.

Its parts: Renal corpuscle, proximal convoluted tubule (PCT), loop of Henle, distal convoluted tubule (DCT). DCT joins the collecting ducts which open into the papilla.

Kidney has an outer cortex and inner medulla.

Cortex

- Covered by capsule.
- Renal corpuscles, greater parts of PCT and DCT located.
- *Subdivided:* Pars radiata [medullary rays (loops of Henle, collecting ducts)] and Pars convoluta (cortical labyrinths).
- Medullary ray and the portions of adjacent cortical labyrinths form a lobule.
- Cortex penetrates into the depth of medulla to form renal columns (column of Bertin).

Medulla

- Partially surrounds the cavity, the renal sinus, opening at the hilus.
- Hilus consists of the ureter with the renal pelvis and the calyces, renal vessels and nerves, loose connective tissue and fat.

- Consists of eight to eighteen medullary pyramids (thin segment of the loop of Henle, collecting ducts).
- Base directed towards the cortex and the apex projects into the minor calyx.
- Two or three pyramids join to form the single papilla.
- Two zones, outer more deeply colored area and inner paler papillary area.

Renal Corpuscle

- Bowman's capsule (parietal layer-squamous epithelium, visceral layer-podocytes) and glomerulus (arterial capillary plexus with afferent and efferent arterioles) form renal corpuscle.
- Have vascular and renal poles.

	PCT	*Loop of Henle*	*DCT*
Features	Longest, most convoluted tubule, forms major portion of cortex	Medulla (pyramids, medullary rays)	Larger lumen, cortex
Cells	• Lined by low columnar or pyramidal cells with brush border • Nuclei round and euchromatic • Granular pink cytoplasm and striated basal region	• *Thin segment:* Lined by low cuboidal or squamous cells • *Thick segment:* Lined by cuboidal cells	• Lined by cuboidal cells devoid of brush border • Nuclei close together, more numerous compared to PCT • Pale staining cytoplasm, less of basal striations

Collecting Tubule

- Initially lined by cuboidal cells, which becomes tall columnar distally.
- Distinguished from convoluted tubules by larger circular lumen, clear lightly staining cytoplasm, distinct cell outlines and absent brush border.

Juxtaglomerular Apparatus

Three types of cells together constitute juxtaglomerular apparatus:

1. Smooth muscle cells in afferent glomerular arteriole highly modified to form the juxtaglomerular cells.
2. Cells in DCT become thin, tall columnar, nuclei closer together appear dark form the macula densa.
3. In between the afferent and efferent arterioles is the presence of the extraglomerular cells (Lacis or mesangial or Polkissen).

Glomerular Filtration Barrier

- Capillary endothelium.
- Fused basal lamina of capillary endothelium and glomerular layer.
- Podocytes of glomerular layer.

Ureter

Mucosa	
• Epithelium	Transitional epithelium
• Lamina propria	Connective tissue with few elastic fibrils, numerous cells, diffuse lymphatic tissue which may take form of lymph nodule
• Muscularis mucosa	Absent
Muscular layer	Inner longitudinal and outer circular layers in the upper 2/3rd and an additional outer longitudinal layer in the lower 1/3rd
Adventitia	Loosely arranged connective tissue with large blood vessels

Urinary Bladder

Mucosa	Thrown into folds
• Epithelium	• Transitional epithelium • *Surface layer:* Dome-shaped cells, intermediate layer: Pear-shaped cells, basal layer: Columnar cells • Epithelium becomes thinner when distended with urine, capable of withstanding osmotic changes, resistant to toxic substances (due to modified areas of plasma membrane called plaques)
• Lamina propria	Loosely arranged connective tissue with lymphocytes and sometimes lymph nodules
• Muscularis mucosa	Absent No distinct submucosa
Muscular layer	Detrusor muscle, inner and the outer longitudinal and the middle circular layers not distinctly differentiated
Adventitia	Attaches the organ to the surrounding structures, consisting of the loosely arranged connective tissue with the blood vessels

CHAPTER

14

Male Reproductive System

The male reproductive system consists of a pair of testes, excretory ducts (straight tubules, rete testis, epididymis, vas deferens, ejaculatory ducts), accessory sex glands (pair of seminal vesicles, prostate gland, pair of bulbourethral glands) and penis. The testes produce sperms and synthesize androgens or sex hormones essential for the process of the spermatogenesis. From the testes the sperm move through the ducts to epididymis for storage and maturation and leaves the epididymis via the ductus deferens and penile urethra.

TESTES

These are the primary reproductive organs or gonads in the male, suspended in the scrotum. Each testis is enclosed in a thick connective tissue capsule, the tunica albuginea; internal to which is a vascular layer of loose connective tissue, the tunica vasculosa. The connective tissue of tunica albuginea posteriorly thickens to form the mediastinum testis. Extending from the mediastinum testis towards the tunica albuginea are the thin fibrous septa that divide the testis into compartments, the testicular lobules. Within each lobule are one to four seminiferous tubules that are not solid and there is intercommunication between lobules. The connective tissue from the tunica vasculosa extends inward into the testis to form the interstitial connective tissue. The interstitial connective tissue with fibroblasts, muscle-like cells, nerves, blood vessels and lymphatic vessels surrounds, binds and supports the seminiferous tubules. Apart from these, in between the tubules are the interstitial cells of Leydig that produce the male sex hormone, the testosterone.

Each seminiferous tubule is lined by complex stratified germinal epithelium containing proliferating spermatogenic cells and nonproliferating supporting or sustentacular cells or Sertoli cells. In the tubules, the spermatogenic cells divide mitotically to form the primary spermatocytes that in turn divide meiotically to form the secondary spermatocytes, which mitotically divide to give rise to the spermatids with haploid number of chromosomes. The spermatids are transformed into sperms by a complex morphological process, the spermiogenesis.

The section of the testis under the scanner (Fig. 14.1) shows the cross-sections of seminiferous tubules. One of the sections shows the plane going through the wall of seminiferous tubule tangentially. In this the lumen is not observed. Seminiferous tubules are surrounded by the connective tissue along with the blood vessels and are lined by complex stratified germinal epithelium.

The sections under low power (Fig. 14.2) and high power (Fig. 14.3) show the tubal epithelium revealing two kinds of cells—proliferating population of spermatogenic cells and nonproliferating population, the sustentacular or Sertoli cells. The Sertoli cells are considerably fewer and recognized by their elongate, pale staining and conspicuous nucleoli. The Sertoli cell cytoplasm extends from the periphery of the tubule to the lumen. The spermatogenic cells consist of successive generations arranged in concentric layers. Thus, the spermatogonia are found at the periphery close to the wall of seminiferous tubule. The primary and secondary spermatocytes lie above them. The primary spermatocytes are the largest population in the seminiferous tubule and are present in the middle of

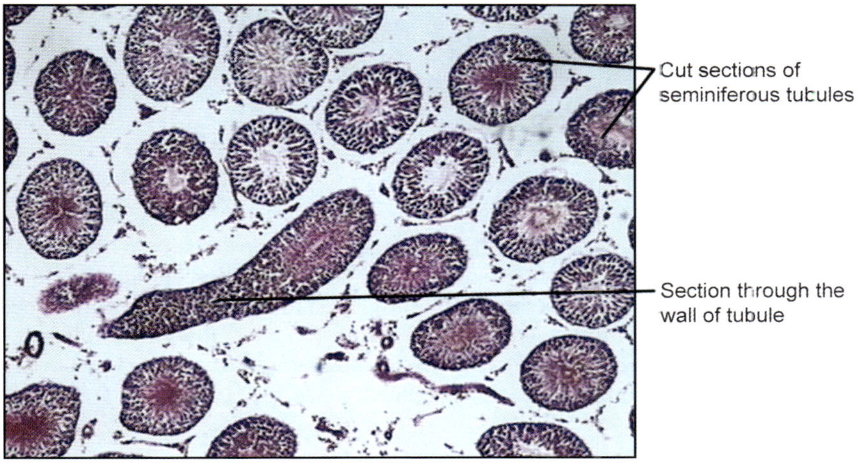

FIGURE 14.1 Testis, H & E, X40

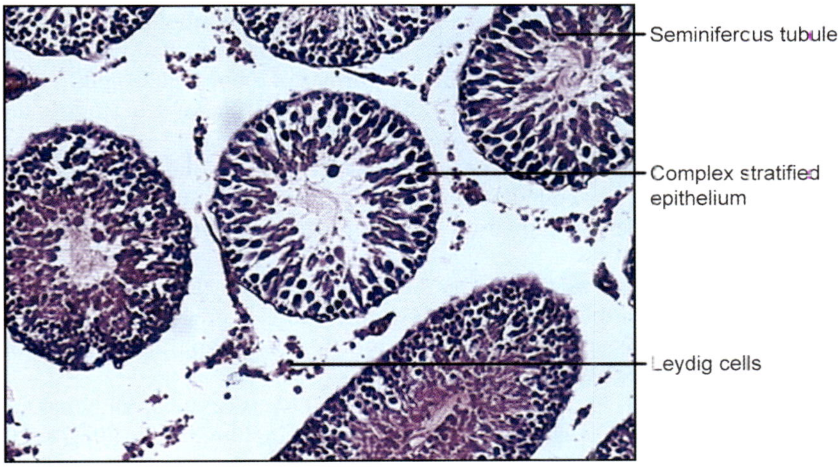

FIGURE 14.2 Testis, H & E, X100

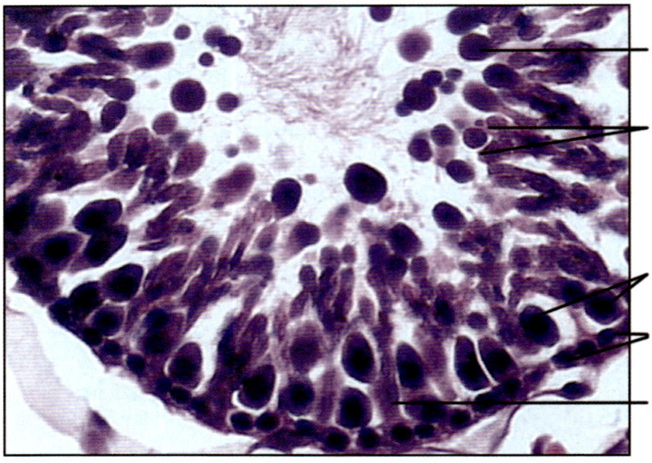

FIGURE 14.3 Testis, H & E, X400

the tubule. The secondary spermatocytes undergo a second meiotic division in a short span of time after their formation and are not frequently seen in seminiferous tubules. The spermatid population consists of one or two generations and occupies the site closest to the lumen. The younger generation of spermatids is composed of round cells and exhibits round nuclei. The interstitial cells of Leydig are conspicuous in the newborn, a reflection of the residual effects of maternal hormones. Leydig cells, however, regress and become conspicuous again at puberty.

EPIDIDYMIS

The epididymis is a crescent-shaped structure that contains the efferent ductules and the duct of the epididymis. It is divided into head, body and tail. The proximal part of head contains ductus epididymis, a single convoluted duct into which the efferent ductules open. The duct is highly convoluted in the head but become less in the body and tail. The epithelium is pseudostratified epithelium with two types of cells, principal cells that are tall columnar and basal cells that are short lying close to the basement membrane. The free surface of the principal cells has stereocilia, the long branching microvilli. Surrounding the epithelial layer is a thin layer of smooth muscle and small amount of connective tissue with blood vessels and nerves.

Section under scanner (Fig. 14.4) shows the highly coiled ductus epididymis. The various shapes of the profiles of the duct reflect its coiled nature. The lumen shows numerous sperms in it and is lined by pseudostratified columnar epithelium. The tubule is surrounded by the smooth muscle and connective tissue.

Section under low power shows (Fig. 14.5) the clear picture of duct of epididymis with its epithelial lining of pseudostratified layer. Darkly stained nuclei are seen. Stereocilia can be appreciated. Numerous sperms are identified in the lumen and the epithelium is surrounded by smooth muscle and connective tissue with cells and fibers.

Section under high power (Fig. 14.6) reveals the two cell types of the epididymal epithelium, the principal cells and the basal cells. Stereocilia, the long branching microvilli extend from the apical surface of the principal cells. The nuclei of the basal cells are spherical and are located in close proximity to the basement membrane, whereas the nuclei of the principal cells are cylindrical

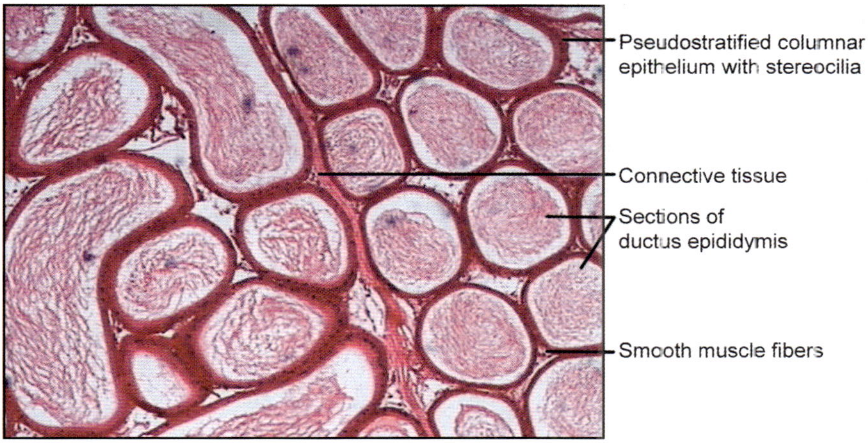

FIGURE 14.4 Epididymis, H & E, X40

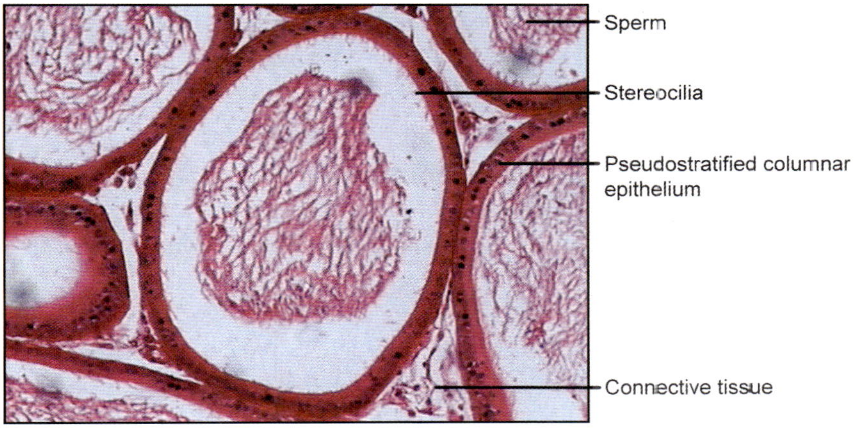

FIGURE 14.5 Epididymis, H & E, X100

and conform to the columnar shape of the cell. Surrounding the duct epithelium is a layer of circularly arranged smooth muscle cells. Adjacent to smooth muscle layer are the cells and fibers of connective tissue with blood vessels and nerves.

DUCTUS DEFERENS OR VAS DEFERENS

The ductus deferens conducts spermatozoa from the epididymis to the urethra. Vas deferens is a thick-walled muscular tube consisting of inner and outer longitudinal layers and a thick intermediate circular layer. Like the distal part of the epididymis, the ductus deferens is innervated by the sympathetic nervous system, producing strong peristaltic contractions to expel its contents into the urethra, during ejaculation. In the terminal part, it joins with the seminal vesicle to form the

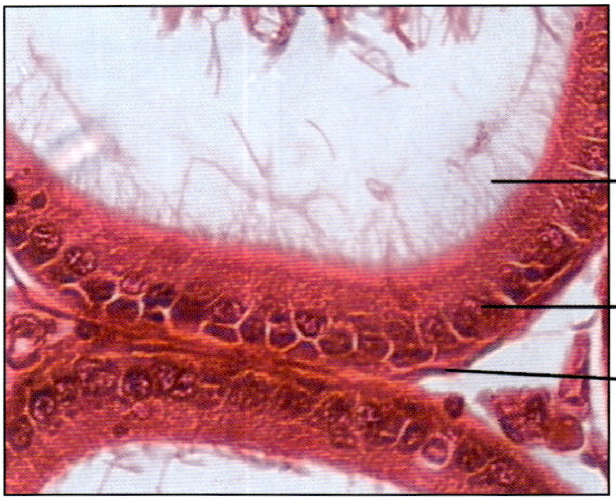

FIGURE 14.6 Epididymis, H & E, X400

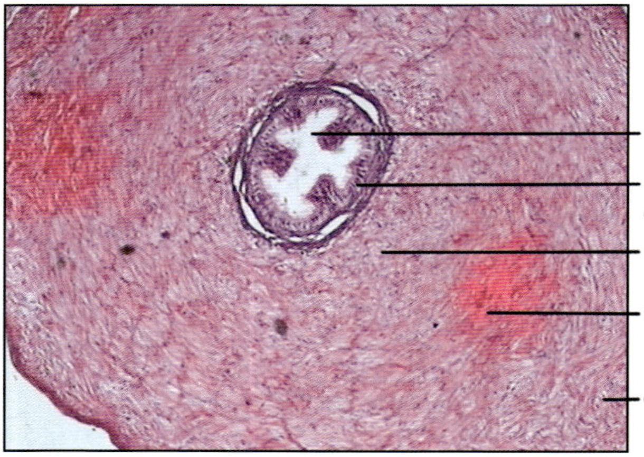

FIGURE 14.7 Ductus deferens, H & E, X40

ejaculatory duct, which pierces the prostate gland and opens into the urethra. The seminal vesicle secretes fructose-rich fluid, the principal metabolic substrate for sperm.

The wall is extremely thick with three layers, the mucosa, muscularis and adventitia. Mucosa is lined by pseudostratified columnar epithelium with stereocilia. The epithelium rests on the lamina propria consisting of loose connective tissue with compact collagen fibers and fine network of elastic fibers. Muscularis, very thick, is arranged in three layers, thick outer longitudinal layer, thick middle circular layer and thin inner longitudinal layer. Surrounding the smooth muscle layer is the adventitia, connective tissue with nerves and blood vessels.

Section under scanner (Fig. 14.7) shows the irregular lumen with thin mucosa, thick muscularis and adventitia. The wall of the ductus deferens is extremely thick, mostly because of the presence

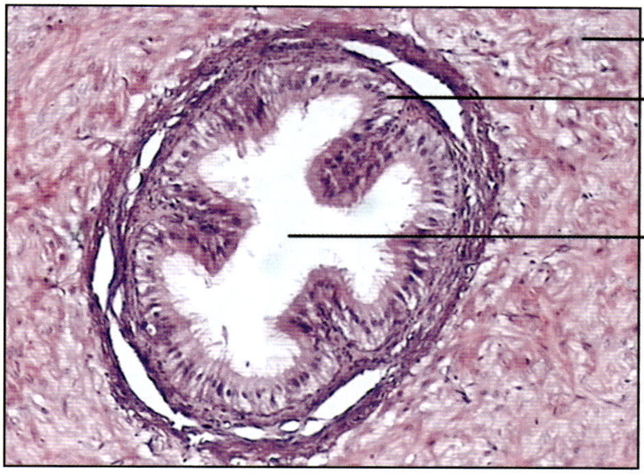

FIGURE 14.8 Ductus deferens, H & E, X100

of a large amount of smooth muscle. The muscle contracts when the tissue is removed, causing the mucosa to form longitudinal folds.

The smooth muscle of the ductus deferens is arranged as thick outer longitudinal layer, thick middle circular layer and thinner inner longitudinal layer. Between the epithelium and the inner longitudinal smooth muscle layer there is a moderately thick cellular layer of connective tissue, lamina propria.

Section under low power (Fig. 14.8) shows the epithelial lining of the ductus deferens consisting of pseudostratified columnar epithelium with stereocilia. It resembles the epithelium of the epididymis, with columnar cells and basal cells. The elongated nuclei of the columnar cells are readily distinguished from the spherical nuclei of the basal cells. The epithelium rests on a loose connective tissue, lamina propria that extends to the smooth muscle. Submucosa is absent.

PROSTATE

The prostate, the encapsulated largest accessory gland of the male reproductive system lies inferior to the neck of the urinary bladder and surrounds the prostatic part of the urethra. The components of prostate are made up of glandular part and fibromuscular stroma. It consists of 30–50 tubuloalveolar glands arranged in three consecutive layers—an inner mucosal layer, an intermediate submucosal layer and a peripheral layer containing the main prostatic glands. The glands of the mucosal layer secrete directly into the urethra; the other two layers have ducts that open into the prostatic sinuses located on either side of the urethral crest on the posterior wall of the urethra. The mucosa of the prostatic urethra is lined by transitional epithelium. The prostatic glands surrounding the prostatic urethra form most of the prostate. The glands are branched tubuloacinar with prostatic concretions, which are solid secretory aggregations of dead epithelial cells and precipitated secretory products, a characteristic feature of the prostate. The glands are lined by pseudostratified columnar or simple columnar epithelium that secretes components of semen. Surrounding the prostatic glands is the fibromuscular stroma with smooth muscle bundles mixed with collagen and elastic fibers.

Section under scanner (Fig. 14.9) shows the tubuloalveolar glands and the fibromuscular tissue that forms the septa between the glandular tissues. Within the lumina various sized prostatic

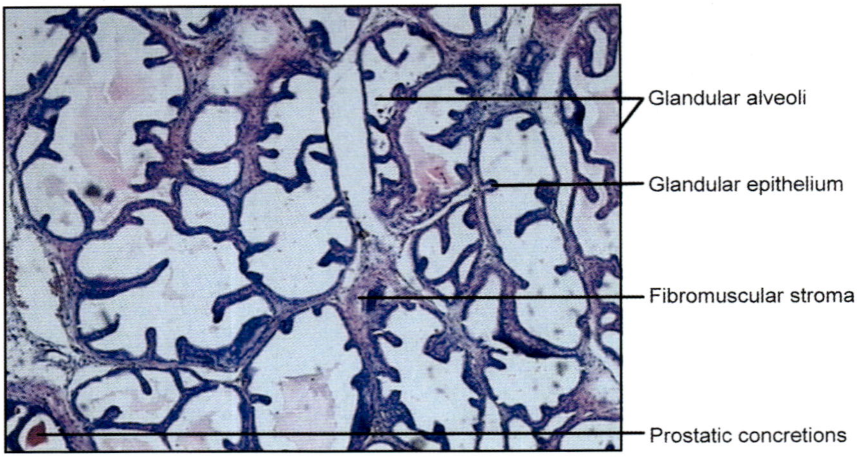

FIGURE 14.9 Prostate, H & E, X40

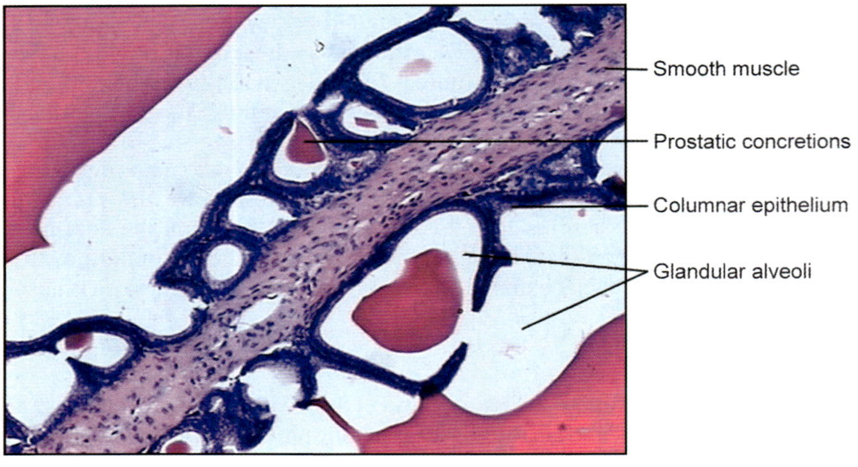

FIGURE 14.10 Prostate, H & E, X100

concretions are seen. The size of the glandular acini is variable. The lumina are irregular and wide because of the protrusion of the epithelium covered with connective tissue. Fibromuscular stroma is observed throughout the gland.

Section under low power (Fig. 14.10) shows the glandular epithelium and some prostatic concretions. Thick fibromuscular stroma is also seen subtending the secretory epithelium of the tubuloalveolar glands as well as in deeper nonsecretory areas.

The section under high power (Fig. 14.11) shows the epithelium and fibromuscular stroma of the alveoli. The glandular epithelium is usually simple columnar or pseudostratified, but in some regions it may be squamous or cuboidal. Aggregations of dead epithelial cells and precipitated

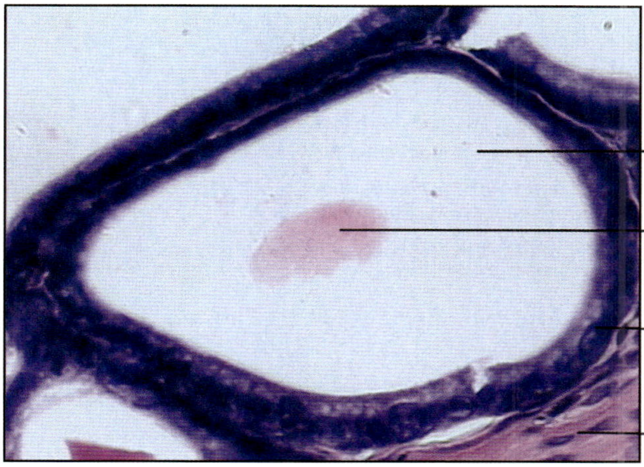

FIGURE 14.11 Prostate, H & E, X400

secretions form prostatic concretions in the lumina of the alveoli and the concretions gradually increase in number and size with age. The concretions stain with calcium salts and thus are easily recognized in X-rays of lower abdomen.

POINTS TO REMEMBER

Testes

Coverings	Tunica vaginalis, tunica albuginea and tunica vasculosa from outwards inside
Division	Divided into lobules consisting of one to four seminiferous tubules
Seminiferous tubule	Epithelium—complicated stratified epithelium of sertoli cells (supporting cells) and different stages of germ cells (spermatogonial cells, primary spermatocyte, secondary spermatocyte, spermatid) Lamina propria/interstitial connective tissue/peritubular tissue—consists of loose connective tissue, blood vessels, lymphatics, interstitial cells of leydig
Blood-testis barrier	Sertoli—Sertoli cell junctional complex

Epididymis

	Single duct highly convoluted
Epithelium	Pseudostratified columnar epithelium consisting of columnar cells with stereocilia and basal cells
Lamina propria	Vascular connective tissue and smooth muscle fibers

Ductus Deferens

Mucosa	
• Epithelium • Lamina propria	Pseudostratified columnar epithelium with stereocilia Loose connective tissue with compact collagen fibers and fine network of elastic fibers
Muscularis externa	Thick smooth muscle layer with two layers, inner circular and outer longitudinal fibers. In proximal part, additional inner longitudinal fibers
Adventitia/Fibrosa	Connective tissue (fibroelastic tissue) with numerous blood vessels and nerves

Prostate

A fibromuscular glandular organ. Stroma and glandular parts, surrounded by vascular capsule of fibroelastic tissue and smooth muscle fibers.

Stroma	Septa penetrate into the prostate from the capsule into the tissue to form the stroma
Glandular part	Compound tubuloalveolar glands divided into three groups—mucosal, submucosal and main prostatic glands Lined by pseudostratified columnar or simple columnar epithelium Ducts lined by columnar epithelium and near the terminal part by the transitional epithelium In some alveoli, spherical bodies, the corpora amylacea are present, which are the condensations of the prostatic secretions (citric acid and acid phosphatase). The number increases with age

CHAPTER

15

Female Reproductive System

Female reproductive system consists of ovaries, uterine tubes, uterus, cervix, vagina, placenta, umbilical cord and mammary glands.

During reproductive life the female reproductive organs exhibit cyclic monthly changes in both structure and function comprising the menstrual cycle. Menstrual cycle is controlled by two pituitary hormones follicle stimulating hormone (FSH) and luteinizing hormone (LH) and two ovarian hormones estrogen and progesterone. The release of the FSH and LH from pituitary is controlled by FSH and LH releasing factors secreted from the neurons in hypothalamus.

The individual organs of female reproductive system perform numerous important functions, the secretion of female sex hormones (estrogen and progesterone), production of oocytes for fertilization, provision of suitable environment for fertilization of oocytes, transportation of embryo to uterus, implantation of embryo, development of fetus during pregnancy and nutrition to newborn.

OVARY

The ovaries are the paired ovoid structures with hilum (for the passage of neurovascular structures) and mesovarium (that joins the ovary to the broad ligament). The functions of the ovary are the production of ova and the synthesis and secretion of estrogen and progesterone. The surface of the ovary is covered by simple cuboidal epithelium, the germinal epithelium overlying the dense irregular connective tissue, the tunica albuginea. Deep to the tunica albuginea is the cortex and medulla, which is highly vascularized. In the cortex are numerous primordial follicles in the connective tissue containing the fibrocytes with collagen and reticular fibers. The primordial follicles are numerous and located near the periphery deep to the tunica albuginea. They are present at the time of birth and remain unchanged until sexual maturation. Squamous layer of follicular cells surrounds oocyte in the primordial follicles. The oocyte that is small in primordial follicle gradually increases in size in primary, secondary and mature follicles. The oogonia are arrested in the prophase of the first meiotic division. At puberty, under the influence of the pituitary gonadotropins, the ovaries begin to undergo the cyclical changes, the ovarian cycle. During each cycle, the ovaries normally produce a single oocyte that is ready for fertilization.

At the beginning of the ovarian cycle, under the influence of the pituitary FSH, some of the primordial follicles begin to undergo changes that lead to the development of a mature

Graafian follicle. These changes include proliferation of the follicular cells and enlargement of the follicles. Although several primordial follicles begin these developmental changes, usually only one reaches maturity and yields an oocyte. Occasionally, two follicles mature and ovulate leading to the possibility of dizygotic twin development. Ovulation is the process of the discharge of the oocyte and its adherent cells. At ovulation, the oocyte completes the first meiotic division and only if fertilization occurs the oocyte completes the second meiotic division. Whether or not fertilization occurs, the other follicles that begin to proliferate in the same cycle degenerate, a process referred to as atresia and these follicles are the atretic follicles.

The primary follicle is small with cuboidal or columnar or stratified cuboidal cells surrounding the oocyte. The secondary follicles are large with antral cavities and situated deep in cortex. Surrounding the follicle are the modified stromal cells, the theca folliculi with two layers, inner theca interna that is secretory layer and outer theca externa, connective tissue layer. The mature follicle has primary oocyte with cytoplasm and nucleus. The wall of the follicle is formed by the granulosa cells surrounded by the theca interna and theca externa. A local thickening of the granulosa cells, the cumulus oophorus projects into the antral cavity like a mound and over it is primary oocyte. The cells surrounding the primary oocyte form the corona radiata. There is the prominent acidophilic staining glycoprotein zona pellucida between the corona radiata and primary oocyte.

Section under scanner (Fig. 15.1) shows the cortex and medulla of the ovary. Single layer of germinal epithelium covers the ovary and is continuous with the serosa of the mesovarium. A dense fibrous connective tissue layer, the tunica albuginea is present under the germinal epithelium and deep to tunica albuginea are the primordial follicles. It is not unusual to see the follicles at various stages of development or atresia. When a primordial follicle begins the changes leading to the formation of a mature follicle, the layer of squamous follicular cells becomes cuboidal and the follicular cells proliferate and become multilayered. The multilayered cells are called the granulosa cells. A follicle undergoing these early changes is called the primary follicle. As the follicular cells increase, small fluid filled spaces arise between them and gradually fuse into a well-defined larger cavity, called the follicular antrum. Now it is called secondary follicle.

The medulla is highly vascular and numerous blood vessels are observed.

Sections under low power (Fig. 15.2) and high power (Figs 15.3A and B) show the different stages of growing follicles. Small follicles identified with no antral spaces between the follicular

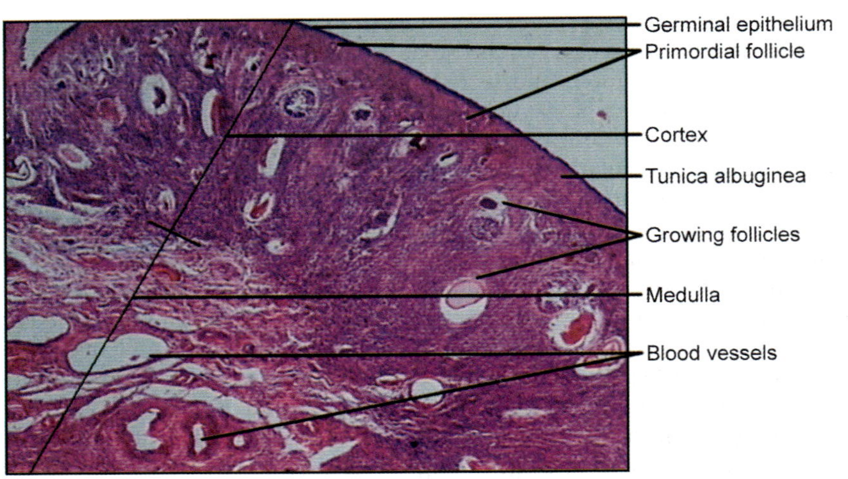

FIGURE 15.1 Ovary, H & E, X40

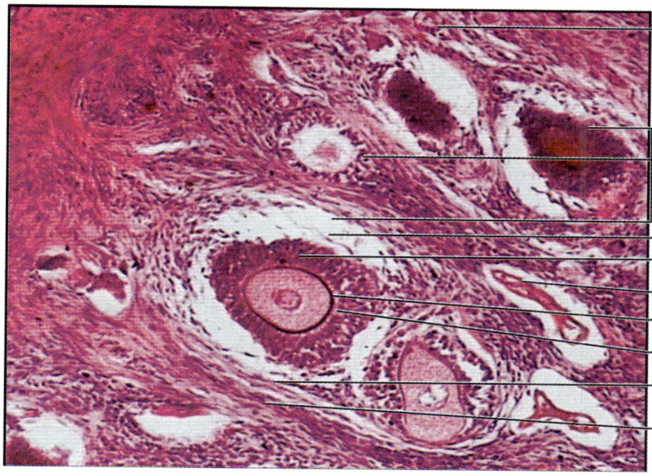

FIGURE 15.2 Ovary, H & E, X100

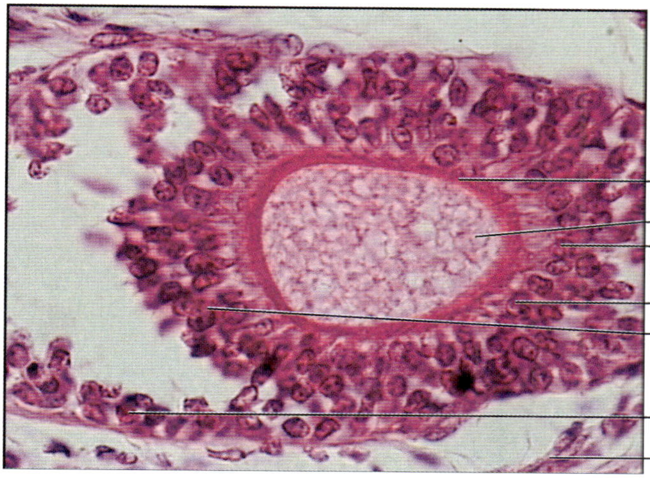

FIGURE 15.3A Ovary, H & E, X400

cells; which can be classified as the primary follicles. In the growing follicles, particularly in the larger follicle with the antrum, the surrounding stromal cells have become altered to form two consecutive layers designated the theca interna and theca externa. The theca interna is more cellular layer and the cells are epithelioid. When seen with the electron microscope the cells display the characteristics of endocrine cells, particularly steroid secreting cells. In contrast, the theca externa is a connective tissue layer. Its cells are more or less spindle-shaped. The antrum is larger and the oocyte is present to one side, surrounded by a mound of follicular cells, the cumulus oophorus. The remaining follicular cells that surround the antral cavity are referred to as membrana granulosa or simply granulosa cells. Atretic follicles are identified by virtue of the retained zona pellucida. In atresia of a more advanced follicle, the follicular cells tend to degenerate more rapidly than the cells

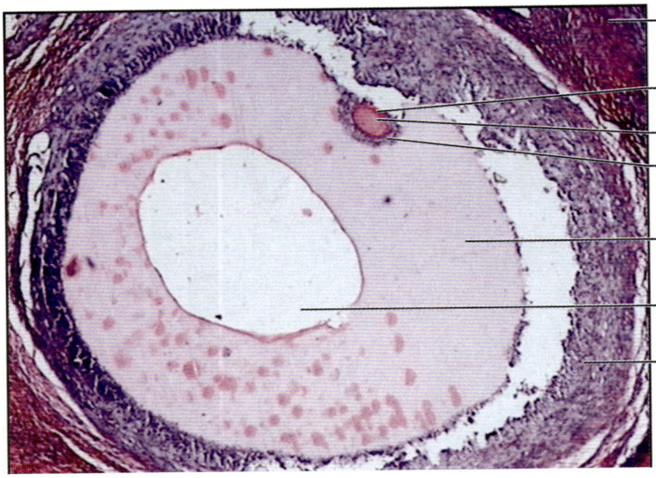

FIGURE 15.3B Ovary, H & E, X400

of the theca interna and the basement membrane separating the two becomes thickened to form the hyalinized membrane, the glassy membrane, which separates an outer layer of remaining theca interna cells from the degenerating inner follicular cells. The remaining theca interna cells may show cytologic integrity. These intact cells remain temporarily functional in steroid secretion.

UTERINE TUBE

Uterine tubes extend from the uterus to the ovaries, where they present an open end called fimbriae for the entry of the ovum, during ovulation. The uterine tubes or the oviducts undergoes cyclical changes along with those of the uterus, but are not pronounced. The epithelial cells increase in height during the middle of the cycle, just about the time the ovum passes through the tube and reduce during the premenstrual period. Some of the epithelial cells are ciliated. The epithelial cells depend on the ovaries for their viability. Not only does the number of ciliated cells increase during the follicular phase of the ovarian cycle, but also removal of the ovaries leads to atrophy of the epithelium and loss of ciliated cells.

The wall of the uterine tube consists of mucosa, muscularis and serosa.

Section under scanner (Fig. 15.4) shows mucosa and muscularis. Many mucosal folds project into the lumen. The lumen extends between the mucosal folds and form deep grooves. The epithelium lining the mucosa is simple columnar epithelium, which has two types of cells, ciliated cells and nonciliated peg cells (secretory). Surrounding the epithelium is the vascularized loose connective tissue, the lamina propria. The muscularis consists of smooth muscle that forms a relatively thick inner layer of circular fibers and a thinner outer layer of longitudinal fibers. The layers are not clearly demarcated, since interstitial connective tissue is abundant. The outermost layer is formed by serosa.

Section under low power (Fig. 15.5) shows the mucosa and muscularis layers. The ciliated cells are identified by the presence of cilia. The nonciliated cells intermixing with the ciliated cells, have elongate nuclei and their apices protrude into the lumen. During secretory phase of menstrual cycle and early pregnancy, the peg cells predominate in the uterine tube. The connective tissue contains cells whose nuclei vary in shape, being elongated, oval or round and are arranged typically

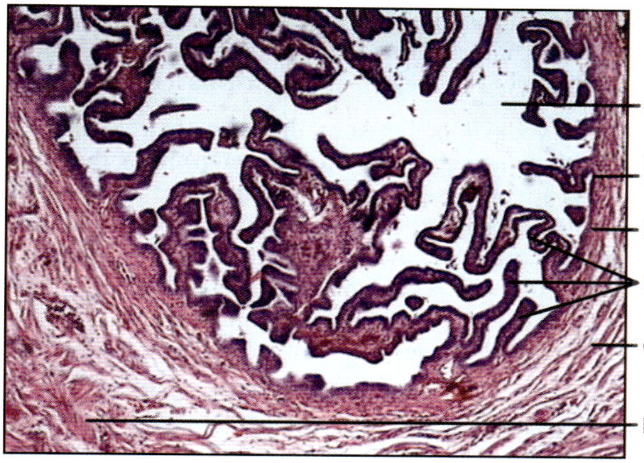

FIGURE 15.4 Uterine tube, H & E, X40

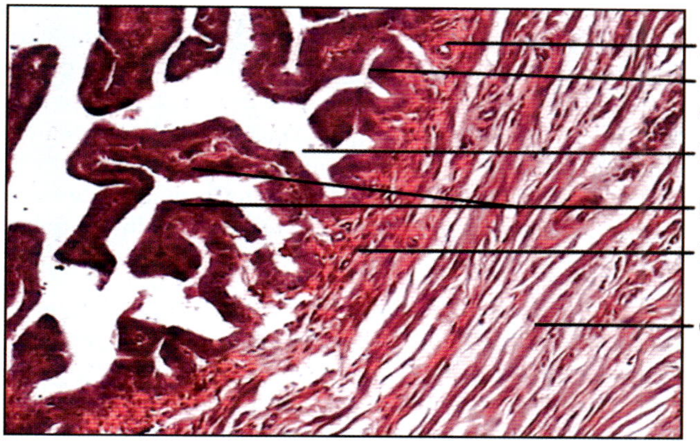

FIGURE 15.5 Uterine tube, H & E, X100

in a random manner. Their cytoplasm cannot be distinguished from the intercellular material. The character of the connective tissue throughout is the same.

UTERUS

The uterus is a hollow, pear-shaped organ with a thick wall and a narrow uterine cavity in the nonpregnant individuals. The uterine wall is composed of mucosa (endometrium), muscularis (myometrium) and serosa or adventitia (perimetrium).

The endometrium is lined by simple columnar epithelium that descends into the lamina propria to form numerous uterine glands. The endometrium has two layers, stratum functionalis and stratum basalis. In a nonpregnant woman stratum functionalis with uterine glands are shed off during menstruation leaving intact basal layer. The myometrium consists of smooth muscle, connective tissue and large blood vessels, that supply the endometrium.

During menstrual cycle, the endometrium exhibits morphological changes that directly correlate with ovarian function. The cyclic changes in nonpregnant uterus are divided into three phases, the proliferative (5–14 days), secretory (15–28 days) and menstrual (1–4 days).

Proliferative phase: After the stratum functionale is sloughed off during menstrual phase, the gland epithelium proliferates and grows over the surface. Below the endometrium is the myometrium, in which a number of large blood vessels are present. Under the influence of estrogen, the various components of the endometrium proliferate, so that the total thickness of the endometrium is increased. The stratum basale remains unaffected by the estrogen. Stratum functionalis increases in thickness and uterine glands elongate and follow a straight course to surface under the influence of ovarian estrogen. The lamina propria in the upper part of endometrium is cellular and coiled arteries are present in the deeper regions of endometrium. The connective tissue layer is more compact and appears darker.

Secretory (luteal) phase: The secretory phase is initiated after the ovulation of the mature follicle. The corpus luteum formed after ovulation secretes estrogen and progesterone, which influence the additional changes occurring in the endometrium. The stratum functionalis and basalis become thicker as a result of increased glandular endometrium and edema in lamina propria. The epithelium of uterine glands undergoes hypertrophy because of increased accumulation of secretory product. The glands become highly coiled and the lumina become dilated with nutritive secretory material rich in carbohydrates. The endometrium in the secretory stage shows numerous shallow sacculations that give the glandular epithelium a serrated appearance. This is one of the distinctive features of the secretory stage. In addition, in this stage, the glandular epithelial cells begin to secrete mucoid fluid rich in glycogen. The product is secreted into the lumen of the glands, causing them to dilate. Typically, the glands of the secretory endometrium are more dilated than those of the proliferative endometrium. The coiled arteries continue to extend into upper portion of the endometrium and become prominent because of the thicker walls.

Menstrual phase: If fertilization of ovum and implantation of embryo do not occur, uterus enters the menstrual phase due to withdrawal of progesterone. The stratum functionalis degenerates and is shed off. The shed endometrium contains fragments of disintegrated stroma (aggregations of erythrocytes that have been extruded from the torn and disintegrating blood vessels, infiltration of lymphocytes and neutrophils), blood clots and uterine glands. The uterine glands and deeper parts of coiled arteries in the stratum basalis remain intact.

The myometrium consists of compact bundles of transverse, oblique and longitudinal section of smooth muscle that are separated by thin strands of interstitial connective tissue with numerous blood vessels. The myometrium also undergoes changes associated with implantation of a zygote. In the nonpregnant uterus, the smooth muscle cells are about 50 micrometers in length, during pregnancy; they undergo enormous hypertrophy, often reaching more than 500 micrometers in length. In addition new muscle fibers develop after division of existing muscle cells and division and differentiation of undifferentiated mesenchymal cells. The connective tissue also increases to strengthen the uterine wall. Fibroblasts increase by division and secrete additional collagen and elastic fibers. After parturition, the uterus nearly returns to its normal size. Most muscle fibers return to its normal size. Some degenerate. The very cells that secreted it, the fibroblasts, digest collagen secreted during pregnancy. Similar, but less pronounced, proliferation and degeneration of fibroblasts and collagen occur in each menstrual cycle.

The perimetrium, the outer serous or visceral peritoneal covering is continuous with pelvic and abdominal peritoneum. It consists of mesothelium and a thin layer of loose connective tissue. The perimetrium covers the entire posterior surface and only a part of anterior surface of uterus. The rest of the uterus is covered by adventitia.

Sections under scanner (Fig. 15.6) and low power (Fig. 15.7) show the endometrium of uterus in proliferative phase and a small portion of myometrium. The glands are slightly wavy in appearance with narrow lumen. The glands are usually straight in the stratum functionale, but may exhibit branching in the deeper portions of endometrium; as a result numerous glands are seen in cross-section. The stratum functionale, which is shed off during menstrual phase, proliferate rapidly under the influence of the estrogens from the remaining intact glands from stratum basale. The glands become long with straight course in stratum functionale to reach the surface. Stratum basale appears the same even under the influence of estrogens. The lamina propria in the upper regions of endometrium is cellular and resembles mesenchyme. The endometrium continues to develop, during the proliferative phase due to the increased levels of estrogen secreted by ovarian follicles. The endometrium reaches the thickness of 3 mm.

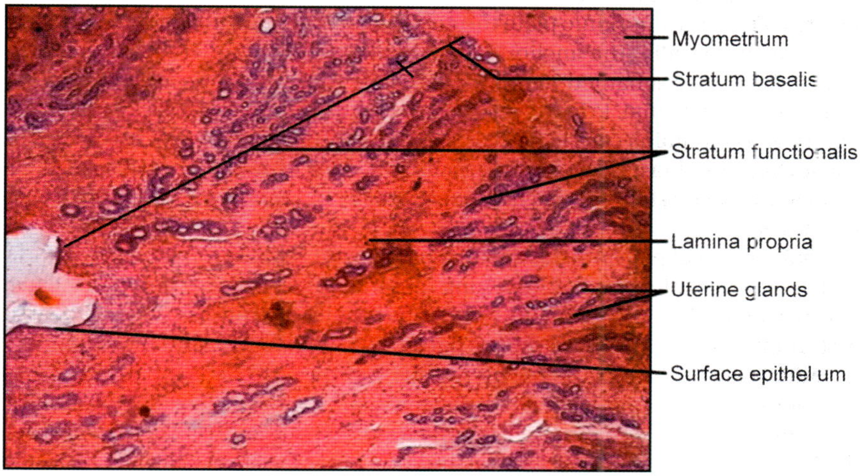

FIGURE 15.6 Uterus, H & E, X40

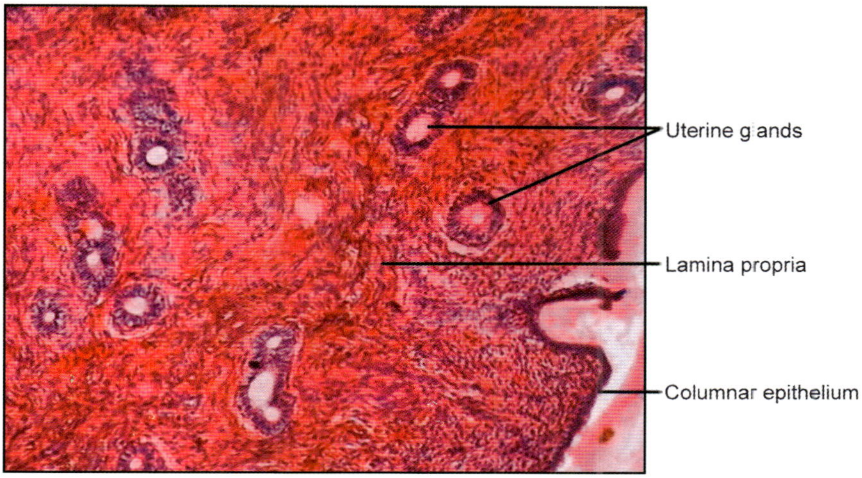

FIGURE 15.7 Uterus, H & E, X100

PLACENTA

The placenta is a disc-like organ that serves the exchange of materials between the fetal and maternal circulations, during pregnancy. One side of the placenta is embedded in the uterine wall at the basal plate. The other side faces the amniotic cavity that contains the fetus. It starts developing immediately after implantation and becomes fully functional after first trimester of pregnancy.

The placenta consists of fetal portion formed by the amnion, chorionic plate, chorionic villi and maternal portion formed by the decidua basalis.

The amnion consists of a layer of simple cuboidal epithelium and an underlying layer of connective tissue. The connective tissue of the amnion is continuous with the connective tissue of the chorionic plate. The chorionic plate is formed by the trophoblast and underlying connective tissue. The connective tissue mass of the chorionic plate is thick and contains the ramifications of the umbilical arteries and vein. The chorionic villi are essential structures for the exchange between mother and fetus. From the chorionic plate the anchoring villi arise and extend to uterine wall and embed in the decidua basalis. The anchoring villi divide to form numerous free villi that float in the intervillous blood spaces bathed in maternal blood. These villi are called floating villi. Three types of villi are seen in placenta. Primary villi—it is formed by cords or masses of cytotrophoblastic cells. Secondary villi—contains central core of mesenchyme surrounded by inner cytotrophoblast and outer syncytiotrophoblast. Tertiary villi—contains core of mesenchyme with blood vessels fibroblasts, macrophage (Hofbauer cells) surrounded by inner cytotrophoblast and outer syncytiotrophoblast.

The maternal portion of placenta has decidua basalis and stratum functionalis of endometrium including fibrin deposits, blood vessels opening into intervillous spaces and uterine glands lying beneath fetal placenta. Below this region is stratum basalis of endometrium with basal uterine glands. The stratum basalis is not shed, during parturition. The decidua basalis contains anchoring villi, large decidual cells and typical connective tissue stroma.

Section under scanner (Fig. 15.8) includes the main substance of placenta, the chorionic villi of different sizes. These emerge from the chorionic plate as large stem villi that branch into increasingly smaller villi. Branches of the umbilical arteries and vein enter the stem villi and ramify through the

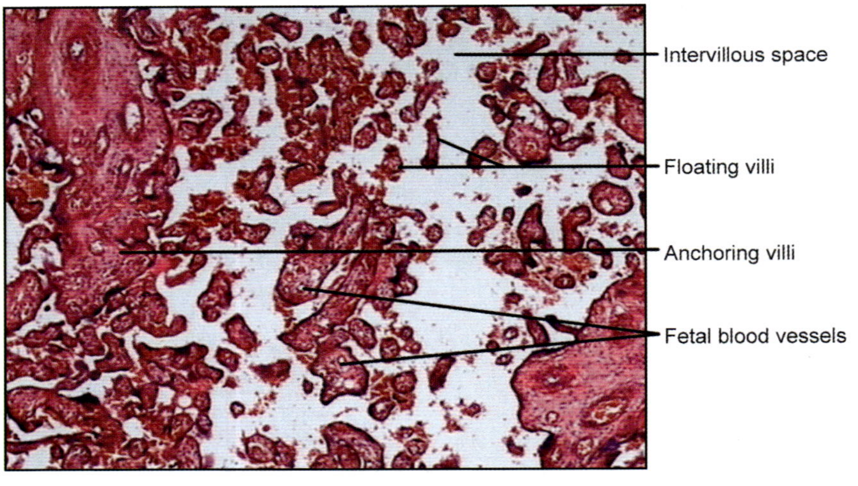

FIGURE 15.8 Placenta, H & E, X40

branching villous network. Some villi extend from the chorionic plate to the maternal side of the placenta and make contact with the maternal tissue and these are the anchoring villi. Other villi, the free villi, simply arborize within the substance of the placenta without anchoring onto the maternal side. Between the villi spaces present are the intervillous spaces.

Section under low power (Fig. 15.9) shows the chorionic villi of different sizes and the surrounding connective tissue. In one of the chorionic villus, fetal blood vessels with connective tissue can be identified. The intervillous spaces with maternal blood cells are observed between the chorionic villi. The outer layer of the chorionic villi, the syncytiotrophoblast can be appreciated.

Section under high power (Fig. 15.10) shows chorionic villi and the surrounding connective tissue. The chorionic villi consist of outer darker staining syncytiotrophoblasts and inner lighter staining cytotrophoblasts. The nuclei of the syncytiotrophoblasts may be more or less evenly distributed, giving the layer an appearance similar to that of cuboidal epithelium. The connective tissue in the villi is identified by the fibers and two types of cells; fusiform fibroblasts and macrophages that are large round having recognizable amount of cytoplasm surrounding the nucleus. The macrophages are considered to be phagocytic and are named Hofbauer cells. Hofbauer cells do not contain any distinctive cytoplasmic inclusions. The connective tissue of the villi contains branches and tributaries of the umbilical arteries and vein. The intervillous spaces contain maternal blood cells.

UMBILICAL CORD

The umbilical cord (Fig. 15.11) connects the fetus to the placenta. It contains two arteries that carry blood from the fetus to the placenta and a vein that returns blood from the placenta to the fetus. The umbilical arteries have thick muscular walls, which are arranged as two layers, the inner longitudinal layer and outer circular layer. Elastic lamellae are poorly developed in these vessels and may be absent. The umbilical vein is similar to the arteries with thick muscular wall. The umbilical vessels are embedded in the mesenchyme consisting of ground substance known as Wharton's jelly. Wharton's jelly is a mass of loose connective tissue with fibroblasts separated by fine collagen fibers and ground substance containing hydrated glycosaminoglycans rich in hyaluronic acid. The umbilical cord is covered by amnion.

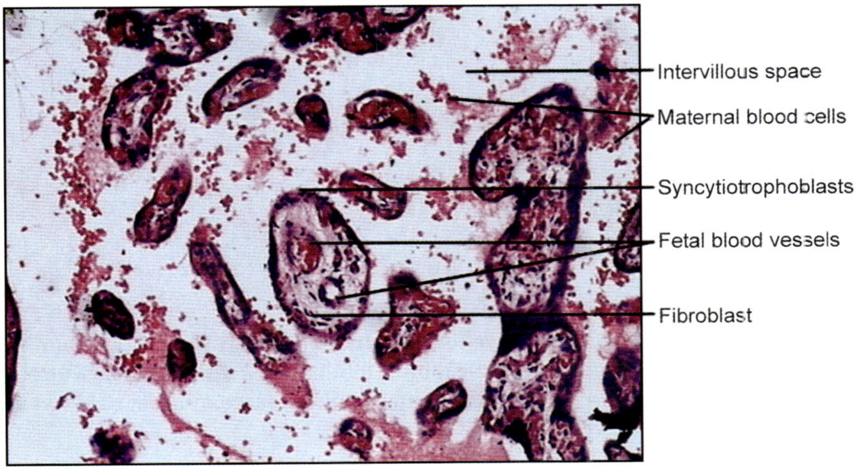

FIGURE 15.9 Placenta, H & E, X100

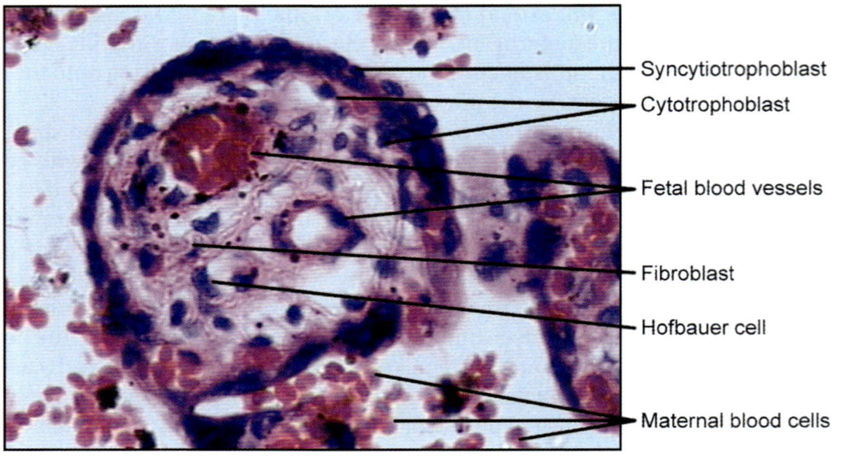

FIGURE 15.10 Placenta, H & E, X400

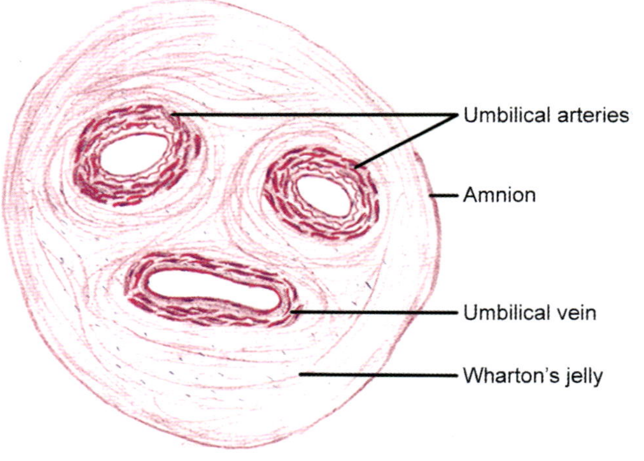

FIGURE 15.11 Umbilical cord, diagrammatic

POINTS TO REMEMBER

Ovary

Covered by the germinal epithelium. Divided into:

- *Inner medulla:* Stroma of loose connective tissue rich in the elastic fibers and blood vessels.
- *Outer cortex:* Cellular stroma containing primordial follicles, Graafian follicles, atretic follicles and corpus luteum and the fibrous tissue with muscle fibers, large number of blood vessels.

Follicles

- *Primordial:* Primary oocyte surrounded by flat cells.
- *Primary:* Primary oocyte with zona pellucida and columnar cells.
- *Secondary:* Primary oocyte with membrana granulosa and antral cavity.
- *Tertiary or Graafian:* Secondary oocyte surrounded by zona pellucida, cumulus oophorus, corona radiata, follicular antrum filled with liquor folliculi, membrana granulosa, theca interna and externa.
- *Atretic follicles:* Follicles degenerate without reaching maturation stage.

Corpus Luteum

- The walls collapse, becomes folded when the follicle rupture.
- Granulosa cells filled with large lipid droplets, yellowish pigment giving the color and form the luteal cells.
- Stroma penetrates into the follicular cells forming the septa.
- Degenerates into a fibrous mass called the corpus albicans, in the absence of fertilization.
- Secretes progesterone.

Uterine Tube

Mucosa	
• Epithelium	Ciliated columnar epithelium and nonciliated peg cells, thrown into numerous irregular folds in infundibulum and ampulla, but decreased towards uterus (isthmus and intramural parts)
• Lamina propria	Rich cellular connective tissue
Muscularis externa	Inner circular and thin outer longitudinal layer
Serosa	Incomplete coat lined by mesothelium

Uterus

Endometrium	
• Epithelium	Simple columnar epithelium
• Lamina propria	Connective tissue with tubular (uterine) glands lined by columnar epithelium and numerous blood vessels. Structure subject to change in accordance with the three phases of the menstrual cycle (proliferative phase, secretory phase and menstrual phase)
• Proliferative phase	Lining epithelium is reformed, endometrium increases in thickness, uterine glands elongate
• Secretory phase	Uterine glands increase in diameter, become tortuous along with blood vessels
• Menstrual phase	3/4th of the endometrium along with entire lining epithelium, uterine glands and blood vessels, is shed off (pars functionalis) leaving behind basal part (pars basalis)
Myometrium	Inner longitudinal, middle circular and outer longitudinal fibers. Muscle cells capable of elongation, new cells also formed during pregnancy
Perimetrium	Serous layer

Placenta

Fetal and Maternal Parts

- *Fetal part:* Consists of chorionic villi (anchoring and floating) arising from the chorionic plate. Spaces between the villi are filled with maternal blood. Villi consist of central core of mesenchymal connective tissue surrounded by cytotrophoblast and syncytiotrophoblast.
- *Maternal part:* Consists of decidua basalis.
- Secretes steroid hormones (progesterone, estrogen), peptide hormones (human chorionic gonadotropin, human chorionic somatomammotropin, human chorionic thyrotropin, relaxin).

Placental Barrier

Until 20 Weeks

Four layers
1. Syncytiotrophoblast
2. Cytotrophoblast
3. Connective tissue of villi
4. Endothelium of fetal capillaries.

After 20 Weeks

Three layers.
1. Syncytiotrophoblast
2. Connective tissue of villi
3. Endothelium of fetal capillaries.

Umbilical Cord

- Two umbilical arteries and one umbilical vein surrounded by the Wharton's jelly and the amniotic layer.
- Primary mesodermal cells of connecting stalk undergo mucoid degeneration and form Wharton's jelly, which protects umbilical vessels.

CHAPTER

16

Endocrine Glands

Endocrine system consists of cells, tissues and organs that synthesize and secrete hormones directly into blood and lymph capillaries. Hence, endocrine glands are ductless glands. The cells in endocrine tissues arranged in cords and clumps are surrounded by extensive capillary network. The hormones released directly into the bloodstream are transported to distant organs and influence the structure and function of target organ cell by binding to specific hormone receptor.

Numerous organs contain individual endocrine cells or endocrine tissues. Pancreas, kidneys, male and female reproductive organs, placenta, gastrointestinal tract are these type of mixed organs. Hypophysis cerebri (pituitary gland), thyroid, adrenal and parathyroid are complete endocrine glands.

HYPOPHYSIS CEREBRI

Hypophysis a compound endocrine gland suspended from the hypothalamus is located in the sella turcica. Hypophysis consists of two major parts, the glandular portion adenohypophysis and neural portion neurohypophysis. Adenohypophysis is further subdivided into pars distalis (anterior lobe), pars tuberalis and pars intermedia. Neurohypophysis is further subdivided into pars nervosa, infundibulum and tuber cinereum. Depending on staining, Pars distalis contains two main types of cells chromophobes and chromophils (acidophils, basophils). Depending on hormonal secretion, five types of cells are classified—somatotrophs (growth hormone), lactotrophs (prolactin), corticotrophs (adrenocorticotropic hormone), gonadotrophs (follicle stimulating hormone, leutinizing hormone), thyrotrophs (thyroid stimulating hormone). Pars nervosa contains unmyelinated axons, supporting cells, the pituicytes and membrane bound neurosecretory vesicles, Herring bodies which contain oxytocin and antidiuretic hormone. Pars intermedia contain follicles, colloid filled cysts and cords of cells that resemble basophils.

Section under scanner (Fig. 16.1) shows part of adenohypophysis, neurohypophysis and pars intermedia. In adenohypophysis cords and clumps of cells with sinusoidal capillaries seen. Pars intermedia contain follicles lined with basophils and colloid filled cysts. Pars nervosa shows unmyelinated axons, Herring bodies and pituicytes with oval nuclei.

Section under low power (Fig. 16.2) shows three parts of the pituitary, the pars distalis, pars intermedia and pars nervosa. The pars intermedia and pars nervosa form the posterior lobe of the pituitary. The pars distalis shows the chromophobes and chromophils with two types of cells, the

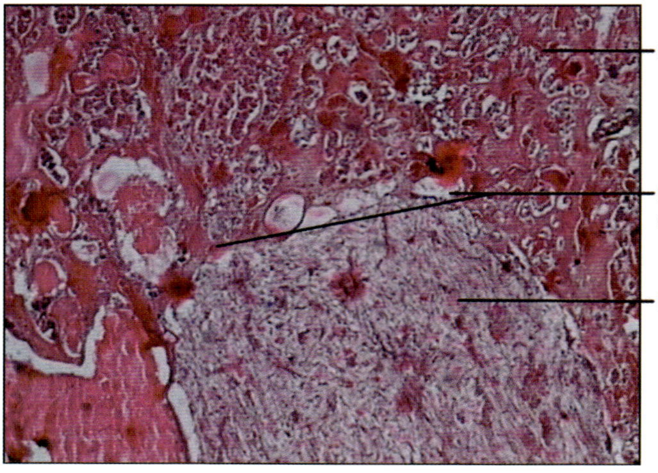

FIGURE 16.1 Hypophysis cerebri, H & E, X40

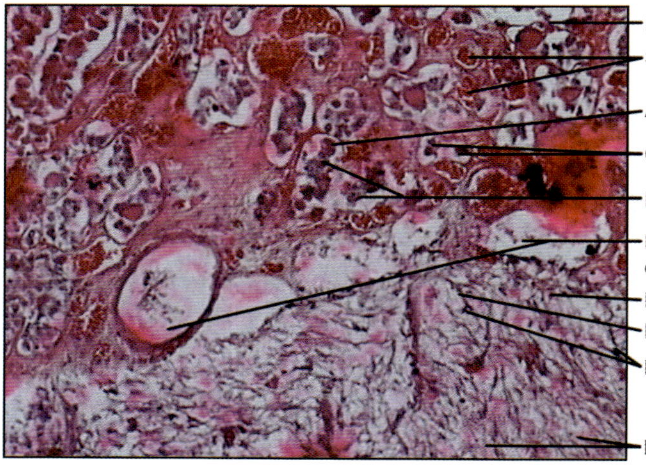

FIGURE 16.2 Hypophysis cerebri, H & E, X100

acidophils and basophils. The pars intermedia situated between the pars distalis and pars nervosa contains follicles and colloid filled cysts. Pars nervosa has unmyelinated axons and the supportive cells, the pituicytes. The cytoplasm of the pituicyte can not be distinguished. The neurosecretory material in pars nervosa is stored in the expanded terminal portions of the nerve fibers as Herring bodies.

Section under high power (Fig. 16.3) shows the details of the cells in the adenohypophysis, chromophobes, and chromophils (acidophils, basophils). In between the cells are present numerous sinusoidal capillaries. The chromophobes are arranged in cords or clumps and the cytoplasm stains poorly in contrast to chromophils because it lacks granules. In between the chromophobes the

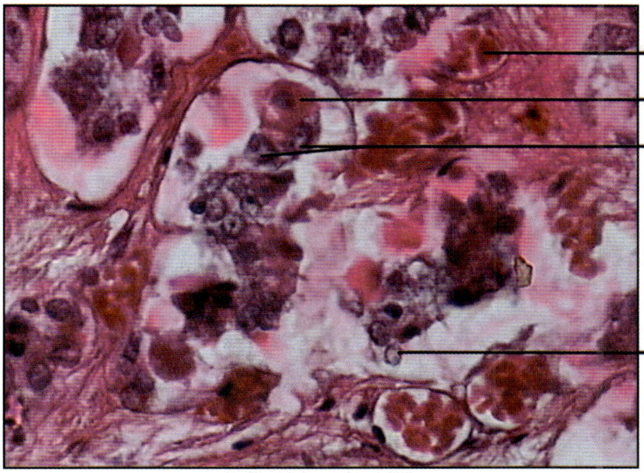

FIGURE 16.3 Hypophysis cerebri, H & E, X400

capillaries are present. The acidophils are identified by the acidophilic staining of the cytoplasm and the basophils by the basophilic cytoplasm. The acidophils and basophils stain deeply because of the secretory granules present in the cytoplasm.

THYROID AND PARATHYROID

Thyroid is single gland consisting of right and left lobes connected in the middle by isthmus. The cells of the thyroid are arranged in spherical structures, the follicles. Follicles are the structural and functional units of thyroid. Each follicle is surrounded by the reticular fibers and vascular network of capillaries that allows easy entrance of thyroid hormone into the bloodstream. The follicular epithelium (follicular cells) can be simple squamous, cuboidal or low columnar, depending on the state of activity of the gland. Follicular cells synthesize, release and store the products outside the cell in the lumen of the follicles as gelatinous substance, the colloid composed of thyroglobulin, a glycoprotein containing several iodinated amino acids. Apart from the follicular cells, pale staining parafollicular cells are also present either in the follicular epithelium (between the basement membrane and the follicular cells) or between the follicles in the connective tissue.

Section under scanner (Fig. 16.4) shows several lobules of the thyroid gland divided by the connective tissue septa extending from the capsule. Different sizes of follicles filled with acidophilic colloid seen in the lobules. It is seen that follicles are lined by simple cuboidal epithelium consisting of follicular cells. Some of them do not show the lumen since they are cut tangentially.

Section under low power (Fig. 16.5) shows the thyroid follicles in detail. The height of the follicular cells depends on their function. In highly active follicles, the epithelium is cuboidal. In less active follicles, the epithelium is flat. Few follicles are filled with colloid some of which show retraction from the follicular wall or distortion because of the slide preparation. A tangential section of the follicle does not show the lumen, but only the cells. Parafollicular cells are located within follicular epithelium between the basement membrane and follicular cells. Parafollicular cells are larger, oval with lighter staining cytoplasm than that of follicular cells and are separated from the lumen by the follicular cells.

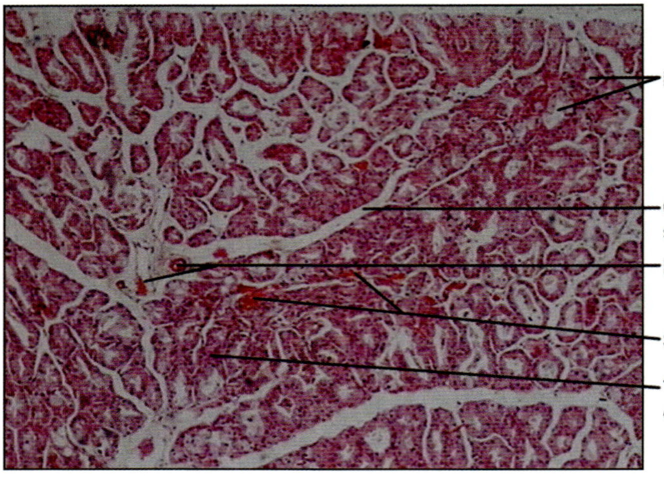

FIGURE 16.4 Thyroid, H & E, X40

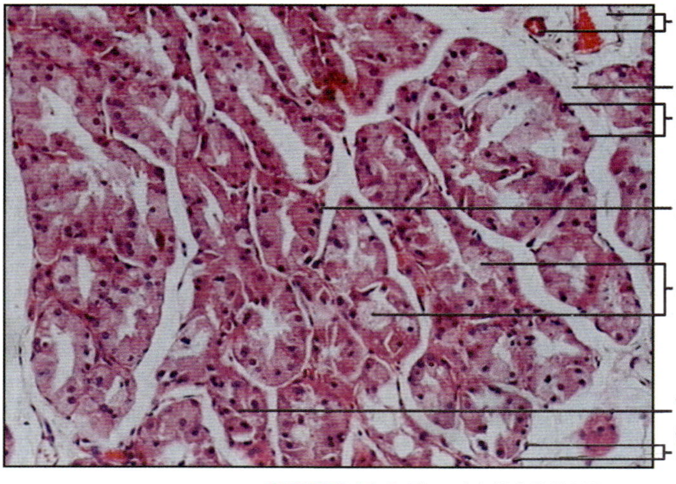

FIGURE 16.5 Thyroid, H & E, X100

Section under high power (Fig. 16.6) shows the retraction of the colloid from the wall of the follicle. The nuclei of the follicular cells are observed clearly. Parafollicular cells identified between the basement membrane and the follicular cells. Sinusoidal capillaries are seen in between the follicles.

Section under scanner (Fig. 16.7) shows parathyroid with a part of thyroid gland.

There are four parathyroid glands. Parathyroids are situated on the posterior surface of the thyroid gland; one on the superior pole and one on the inferior pole of each lobe; but are separated from the thyroid by thin connective tissue capsule. Cells are arranged in cords or clumps surrounded by rich network of capillaries. Two types of cells are present in parathyroid gland, the chief cells and

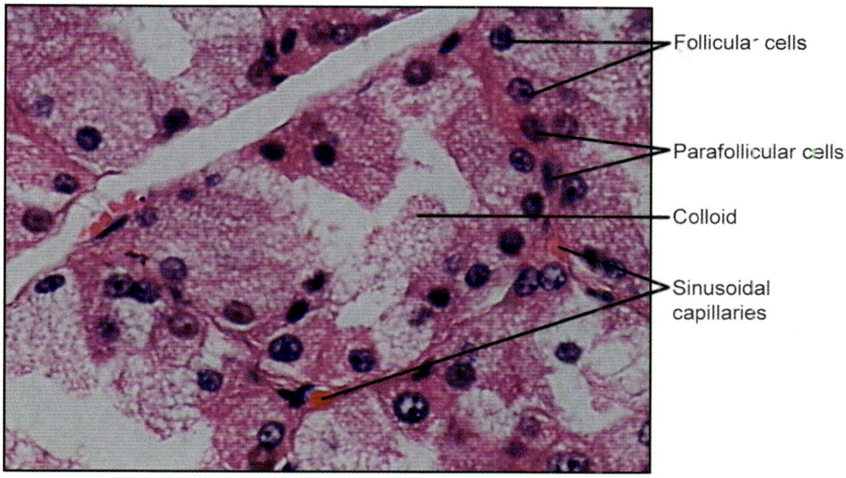

FIGURE 16.6 Thyroid, H & E, X400

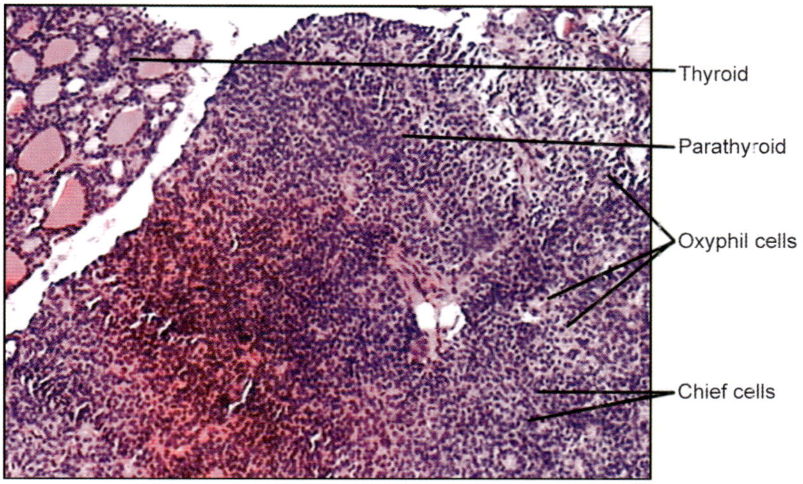

FIGURE 16.7 Parathyroid, H & E, X40

oxyphil cells. Chief cells most numerous are round and have pale lightly acidophilic cytoplasm. They secrete parathormone. Oxyphil cells are larger, found in small groups or in single and are less numerous than chief cells and exhibit acidophilic cytoplasm with smaller, darker staining nuclei.

ADRENAL GLAND

Adrenal glands are present at the superior pole of each kidney. Each gland is surrounded by dense irregular connective tissue capsule and is embedded in adipose tissue around the kidneys. Each gland consists of the outer cortex and inner medulla. The cortex and medulla have distinct

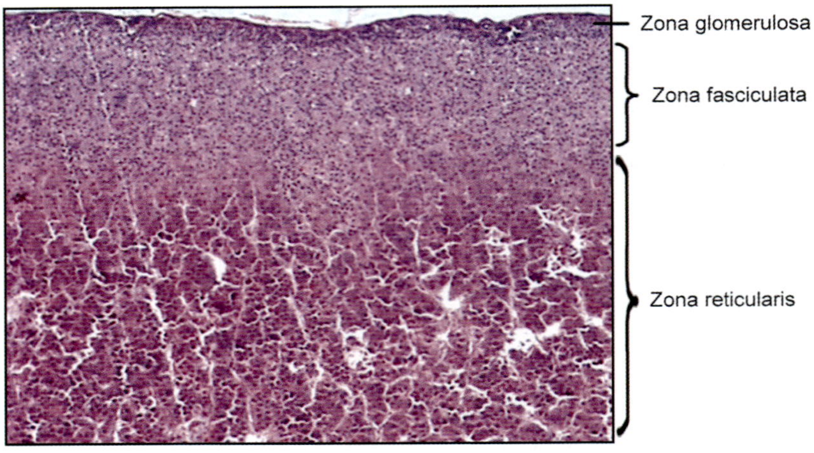

FIGURE 16.8 Adrenal gland, cortex, H & E, X40

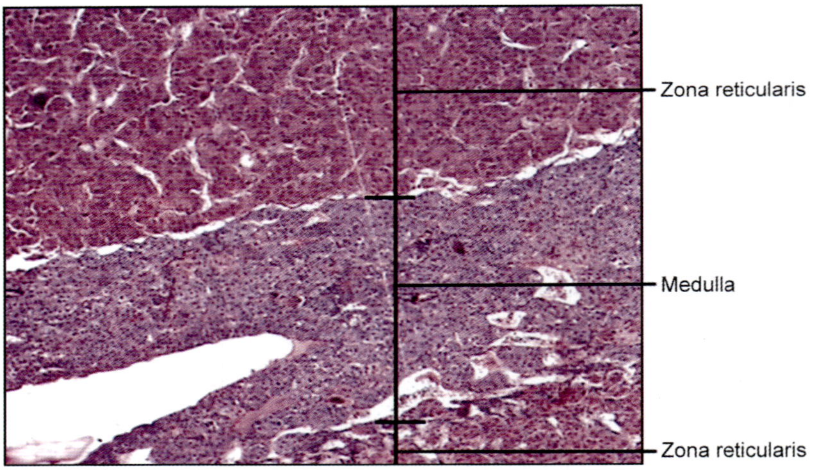

FIGURE 16.9 Adrenal gland, medulla, H & E, X40

embryologic origins, structures and functions, but are located in one organ and have common blood supply.

The adrenal cortex has three concentric layers, the zona glomerulosa, zona fasciculata and zona reticularis. Zona glomerulosa is a thin zone deep to capsule and cells are arranged in small clumps. Zona fasciculata is the middle layer thickest of all with cells arranged in vertical columns (two cell thickness) adjacent to straight capillaries. Zona reticularis innermost layer adjacent to adrenal medulla has cells arranged in cords or clumps. The cells in cortex produce three types of steroid hormones, the mineralocorticoids by zona glomerulosa, glucocorticoids by zona fasciculata and sex hormones by zona reticularis.

Medulla present in the center of the gland has cells arranged in small cords, which are modified postganglionic sympathetic neurons, synthesize and secrete catecholamines.

Section under scanner (Figs 16.8 and 16.9) shows the three layers of cortex and medulla. A thick connective tissue capsule covers the cortex. The sinusoidal capillaries are found throughout the gland. The three layers of the cortex are zona glomerulosa under the connective tissue capsule, middle zona fasciculata and adjacent to adrenal medulla is the zona reticularis.

Section under low power (Fig. 16.10) shows the arrangement of the cells in zona glomerulosa and zona fasciculata. A part of the zona reticularis is observed. Zona glomerulosa is present at the outer part under the capsule. Cells are arranged in ovoid groups and the cytoplasm of these cells contains few lipid droplets. Cells in zona fasciculata are arranged in columns or radial plates and

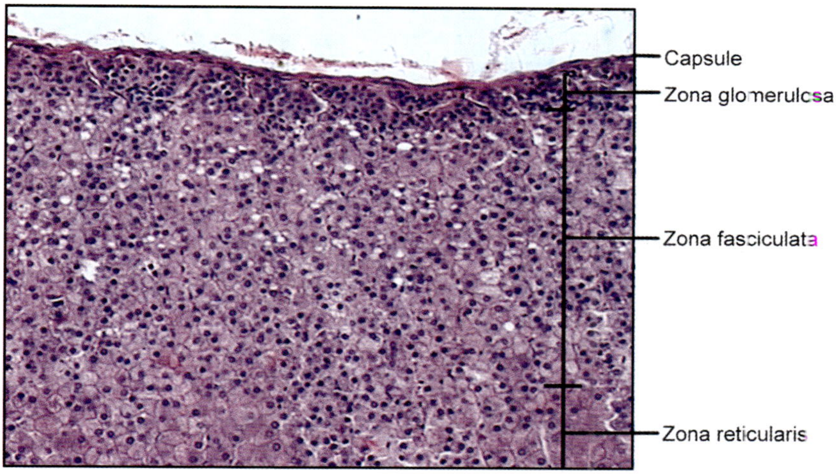

FIGURE 16.10 Adrenal gland, H & E, X100

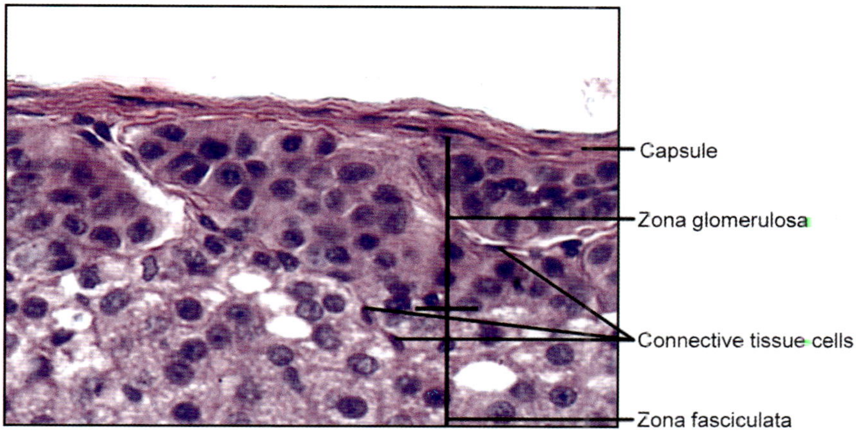

FIGURE 16.11 Adrenal gland, H & E, X400

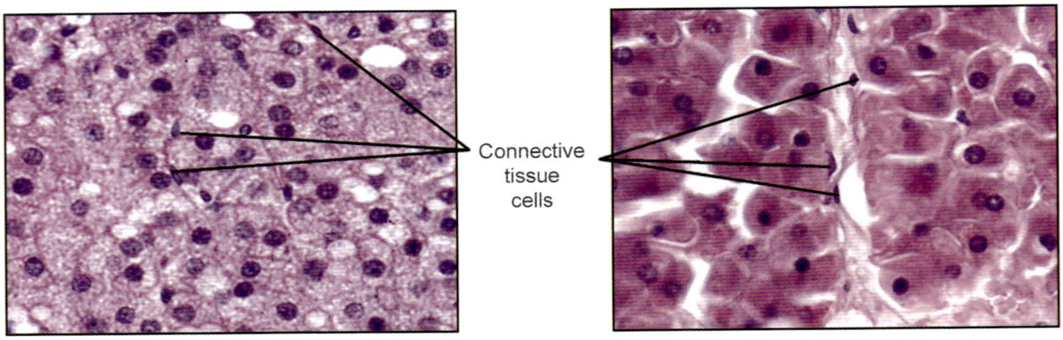

FIGURE 16.12 Adrenal gland, zona fasciculata and zona reticularis, H & E, X400

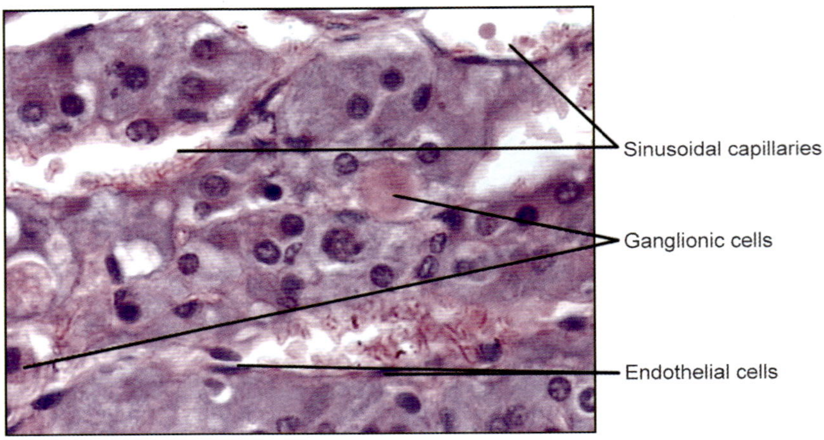

FIGURE 16.13 Adrenal gland, medulla, H & E, X400

appear vacuolated because of the increased lipid in the cytoplasm. Cells in the zona reticularis form anastomozing cords and often contain the dark staining lipofuscin pigment.

Cells in the medulla show clear cytoplasm and the sinusoidal capillaries drain the contents of medulla into the medullary veins.

Sections under high power (Figs 16.11 to 16.13) show the cells in different parts of cortex and medulla. The small cells in the zona glomerulosa are arranged in cords or clumps. The nuclei of these cells are spherical and the cytoplasm stains lightly. Because of the less amount of cytoplasm, the nuclei appear crowded. The cells in zona fasciculata are arranged in sheets of two cells width. The nuclei are same as those of zona glomerulosa or slightly larger that are arranged at a distance from each other. The cytoplasm is more and gives a spongy appearance, due to lipid droplets. Binucleate cell can be observed in this region. The cells of zona reticularis are small and arranged as interconnecting, irregular cords and sheets. The capillaries between the cells appear dilated as compared to the other parts of the cortex. Between the cells of the cortex are elongated nuclei of connective tissue cells or endothelial cells of capillaries. The adrenal medulla consists of large cells arranged as short interconnecting cords surrounded by blood vessels. Numerous membrane bound granules are present in the cells.

POINTS TO REMEMBER

Pituitary Gland

Adenohypophysis	Pars anterior or pars distalis, pars intermedia and pars tuberalis
Pars anterior	75% of the gland. The parenchyma is formed by anastomozing cords of cells and sinusoidal capillaries. The cells are of two categories
• Chromophobes (50%)	No affinity for usual dyes, present in the central part, pale staining cytoplasm, cell boundaries not clear
Chromophils (50%)	
• Acidophils (40%)	Based on the staining, two types of cells identified. Predominate in the periphery. Larger cells with cytoplasm having secretory granules. Based on secretory nature subdivided into somatotrophs and mammotrophs
• Basophils (10%)	Present in the center. Cytoplasm contains basophilic granules of irregular size. Based on the secretory nature, subdivided into gonadotrophs, thyrotrophs and corticotrophs
Pars intermedia	Rudimentary in humans and is made of basophilic cells and small vesicles that often contain colloid
Pars tuberalis	Surrounds the infundibulum of neurohypophysis and highly vascular. Cells arranged in cords along the sides of blood vessels. Primarily have basophilic cells with few chromophobes
Neurohypophysis	• Pars nervosa and infundibulum. • Unmyelinated axons extending from secretory neurons present in hypothalamus reach pars nervosa and infundibulum, forming the hypothalamohypophyseal tract and tuberoinfundibular tract. • Also consists of connective tissue cells and specific type of cells called pituicytes. • Axons dilated in terminal parts closely related to blood capillaries and are surrounded by neurosecretory granules, bounded by a membrane. These accumulations are called as Herring bodies. Stores oxytocin and vasopressin secreted in hypothalamus.

Thyroid Gland

Follicles and pink stained colloid in the lumen of the follicles are seen.

- Structural unit of thyroid is the follicle (acinus).
- Covered by loose connective tissue capsule, sends septa into parenchyma, which become thinner and reaches all follicles.
- Cells vary in size depending on the state of activity.
- *Moderately active:* Simple cuboidal epithelium, enclose cavity filled with colloid.
- *Highly active:* Columnar epithelium, scanty colloid.
- *Inactive:* Flat squamous epithelium, follicle distended with abundant colloid.
- Secretes T3 and T4.

- In between the follicular cells and basement membrane are some pale staining cells, the parafollicular cells (C-cells), which secrete calcitonin.

Adrenal Gland

Covered by a capsule of dense collagenous connective tissue and is divided into two regions, cortex and medulla.

Cortex

Three concentric layers.

	Zona glomerulosa	*Zona fasciculata*	*Zona reticularis*
Location	Beneath the capsule	Middle layer	Adjacent to medulla
Cells	Cells arranged in rounded clumps surrounded by capillaries	Cells arranged in straight cords, one or two cells thick, running at right angles to the surface, with the sinusoids between them	Cells arranged in closely packed irregular cords forming an anastomozing network. Cells smaller than the other two zones
Secretion	Mineralocorticoids involved in maintenance of electrolyte and water balance	Glucocorticoids, concerned with regulation of carbohydrates, protein and fat metabolism. Produce estrogen and androgen in small amounts	Secretion same as the zona fasciculata

Medulla

- Closely-packed clumps of polyhedral epitheloid cells arranged in cords.
- Supported by fine collagenous network containing numerous capillaries and venules, which drain blood from sinusoids of cortex.
- Secrete catecholamines, adrenaline and noradrenaline under the control of sympathetic nervous system.

CHAPTER

17

Eye

The eye is a highly specialized organ, with protective covering to maintain the shape, lens for focusing, photosensitive cells (rods and cones) to respond to light stimuli, numerous cells to process the visual information and nerves to conduct the information to the brain.

The eyeball has three layers, outer fibrous layer (sclera, cornea), middle vascular layer uvea (choroid, ciliary body, iris) and inner nervous layer (retina). The sclera composed of collagen fibers is opaque and forms two-thirds of the fibrous layer and anteriorly continues with the transparent cornea through which light rays enter the eye. The junction between the sclera and cornea is the limbus. The choroid and ciliary body are present deep to the sclera The choroid has numerous blood vessels that nourish the structures in the eyeball. The ciliary body is composed of smooth ciliary muscle and the ciliary processes. The iris partially covers the lens and surrounds the opening, the pupil. The retina is photosensitive where cells are stimulated by light. In the posterior part of the eye is a small yellow-pigmented spot, the macula lutea with a central shallow depression, the fovea. The fovea is devoid of rods and blood vessels, but contains only cones. The part where the optic nerve leaves the eyeball is the optic disc or optic papilla, which lacks both rods and cones and forms the blind spot of the eye. The eye has three chambers, anterior chamber between the cornea and iris, posterior chamber between the iris and lens, vitreous body between the lens and retina. The anterior and posterior chambers are filled with watery fluid, the aqueous humor and the large vitreous body is filled with gelatinous material, the transparent vitreous humor.

CORNEA

Cornea is avascular, transparent and forms the refractive layer of the eye that is covered by stratified nonkeratinized squamous epithelium. The cornea consists of five layers, the corneal epithelium, anterior limiting membrane, substantia propria, posterior limiting membrane and corneal endothelium. Corneal epithelium is formed by the stratified squamous nonkeratinized epithelium, where the basal layer is columnar resting on thin basement membrane. Intermediate layers are formed by polygonal cells and surface layers by squamous cells. Anterior limiting membrane (Bowman's membrane) is a thick homogeneous layer, which supports the basement membrane of corneal epithelium. The stroma in substantia propria consists of alternating lamellae of type II collagen fibrils and fibroblasts. The fibrils in each lamella are extremely uniform in diameter and uniformly spaced, fibrils in adjacent lamellae are arranged at right angles to each other. The regular arrangement of fibrils is responsible for the transparency of cornea. The single layer of low cuboidal cells (corneal endothelium or posterior epithelium) line the posterior surface that rests on the thickened basal lamina, the posterior limiting membrane (Descemet's membrane). The metabolic exchange of avascular cornea occurs through the corneal endothelium.

Section under scanner (Fig. 17.1) shows the five layers of the cornea. The corneal epithelium presents a uniform thickness and the underlying stroma has a homogeneous appearance. The white spaces seen are the artifacts occurred, during tissue preparation. The corneal epithelium lies on the basement membrane, the anterior limiting membrane (Bowman's membrane). The corneal endothelium lies on the Descemet's membrane, which is not clear in the picture.

Section under low power (Fig. 17.2) shows the full thickness of cornea in detail. The cells of the epithelial layer are clearly appreciated. The basal layer formed by the columnar cells rests on the Bowman's membrane. Nuclei of the fibroblasts of the stroma lying between lamellae observed.

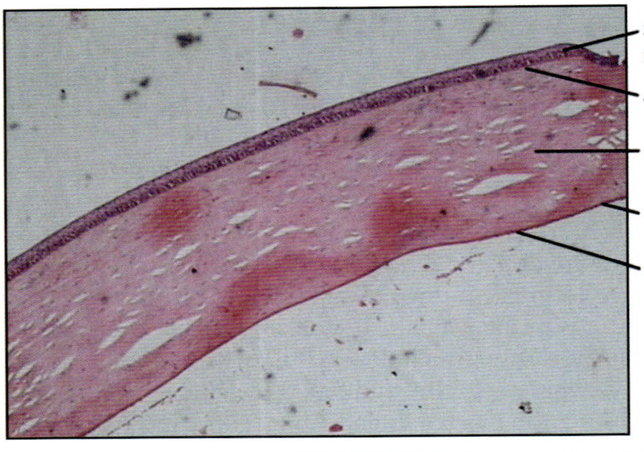

FIGURE 17.1 Cornea, H & E, X40

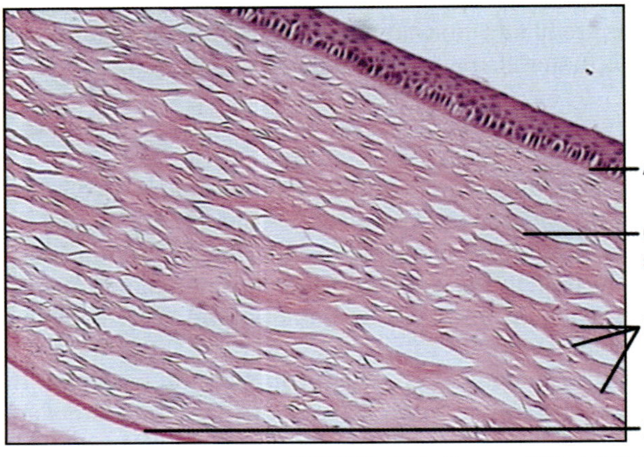

FIGURE 17.2 Cornea, H & E, X100

The posterior surface of the cornea is lined by a simple squamous epithelium, the corneal endothelium lying on thick posterior basement membrane, the Descemet's membrane.

Sections under high power (Figs 17.3A and B) show the corneal epithelium and corneal endothelium clearly. The corneal epithelium has three layers and cells, the basal layer formed by the columnar cells, middle layer by the polyhedral cells and superficial cells by the squamous cells. The thick homogeneous appearing Bowman's membrane can be appreciated deep to the columnar cells. Note the stromal tissue having a homogeneous appearance, that is a reflection of the dense packing of collagen fibrils. On the posterior surface the corneal endothelium formed by squamous cells are well-appreciated with the Descemet's membrane.

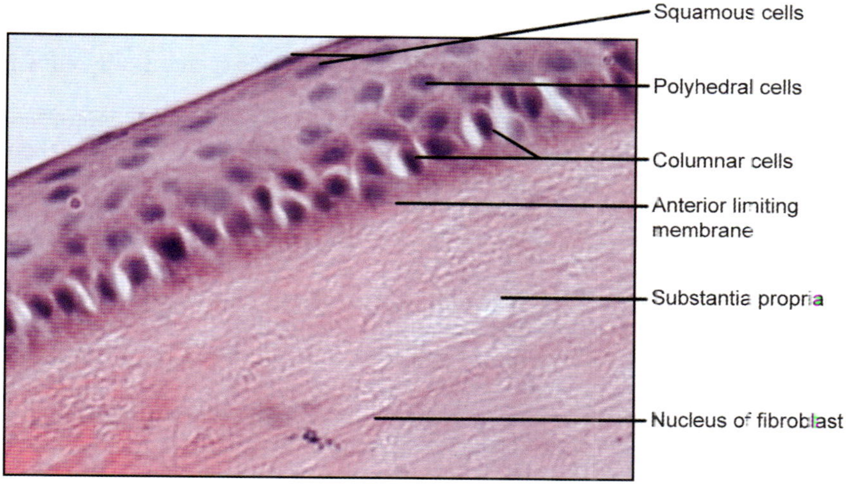

FIGURE 17.3A Cornea, H & E, X400

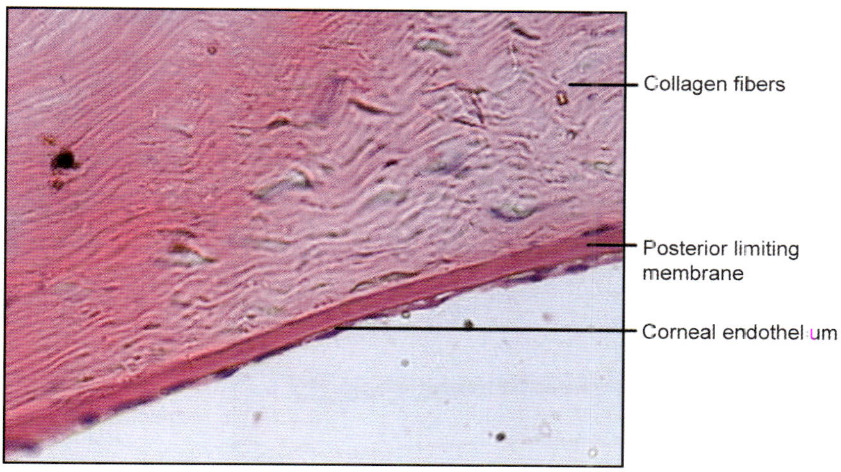

FIGURE 17.3B Cornea, H & E, X400

RETINA

The retina is the projection of the forebrain and is a multilayered structure consisting of photoreceptors, some of which are specialized as conducting and associating neurons and supporting cells (Müller's cells). External to the neural retina is a layer of simple columnar epithelium. The Müller's cells are comparable to neuroglia in the rest of the central nervous system. The processes of Müller's cells ramify through the entire thickness of the retina. The internal limiting membrane is the basal lamina of these cells. The external limiting membrane is actually a line formed by the junctional complexes between the processes of these cells and the photoreceptor cells.

The neurons of the retina are arranged sequentially in three layers, the deep layer of rods and cones, intermediate layer of bipolar, horizontal and amacrine cells and superficial layer of ganglion cells.

On the basis of structural features that are evident in histologic sections, the retina is divided into ten layers, from posterior to anterior (Figs 17.4 to 17.6).

1. Retinal pigment epithelium, the outermost layer is not part of the neural part of retina, but is associated with it. The basement membrane forms the innermost layer of glassy membrane of choroid. The cuboidal cells contains melanocytes and the cytoplasmic processes with pigment granules extend between rods and cones.
2. Layer of rods and cones, the photoreceptor layer of the retina. The rods are slender and cones are thick.
3. External limiting membrane, a line formed by the junctional complexes of the photoreceptor cells, along with the processes of Müller's cells.
4. Outer nuclear layer contains nuclei of rod and cone cells and the outer processes of Müller's cells.
5. Outer plexiform layer contains neural processes and synapses of rod and cone cells with bipolar, amacrine, interplexiform and horizontal cells.

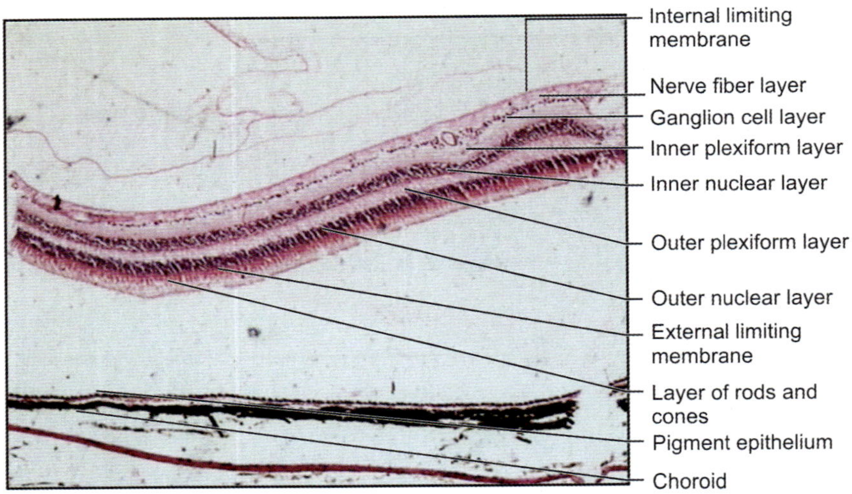

FIGURE 17.4 Retina, H & E, X40

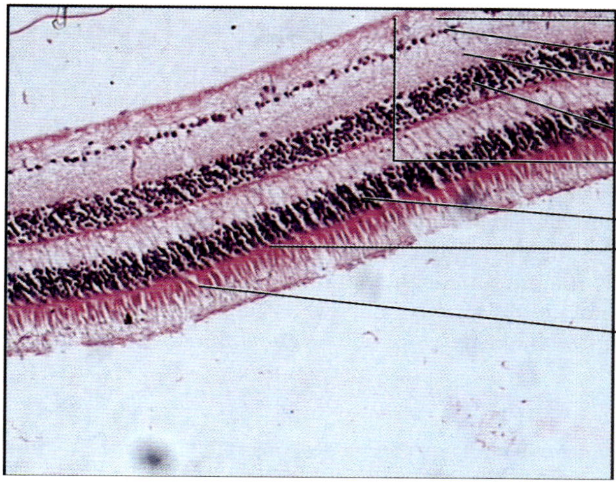

FIGURE 17.5 Retina, H & E, X100

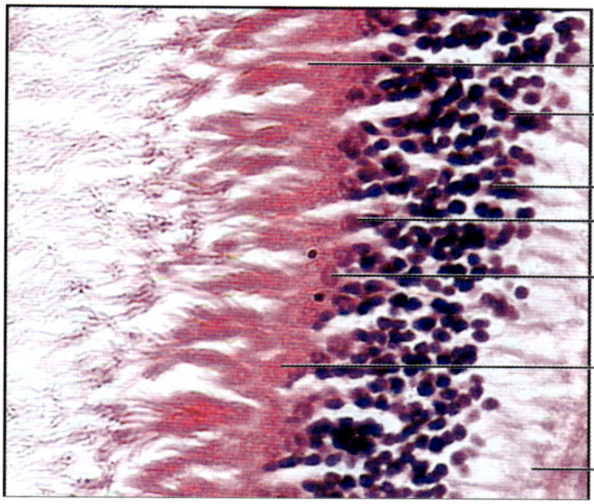

FIGURE 17.6 Retina, H & E, X400

6. Inner nuclear layer contains nuclei of bipolar, horizontal, interplexiform, amacrine and Müller's cells.
7. Inner plexiform layer contains processes and synapses of bipolar with horizontal, interplexiform, amacrine and ganglion cells.
8. Layer of ganglion cells contains cell bodies and nuclei of ganglion cells and Müller's cells.
9. Nerve fiber layer contains axons of ganglion cells, which converge towards optic disc to form the optic nerve and the inner fibers of Müller's cells.
10. Internal limiting membrane consists of the terminations of inner fibers of Müller's cells.

OPTIC NERVE

The optic nerve, the nerve of vision is made up of myelinated nerve fibers. The site where the optic nerve leaves the eyeball is the optic disc, which is characteristically marked by a depression. Receptor cells are not present at the optic disc and because it is not sensitive to light stimulation, it is referred to as the blind spot. The fibers that give rise to the optic nerve originate in the retina, more specifically, in the ganglion cell layer. They traverse the sclera through a number of openings to form the optic nerve. The region of the sclera that contains these openings is called the lamina cribrosa or the cribriform plate. After piercing the lamina cribrosa, the nerve fibers become myelinated. It is covered by meninges, namely the dura mater, arachnoid mater and pia mater. The dura mater is of tough consistency and made up of dense connective tissue. The arachnoid mater forms the middle layer. It is made up of cobweb like network of delicate connective tissue. The pia mater is

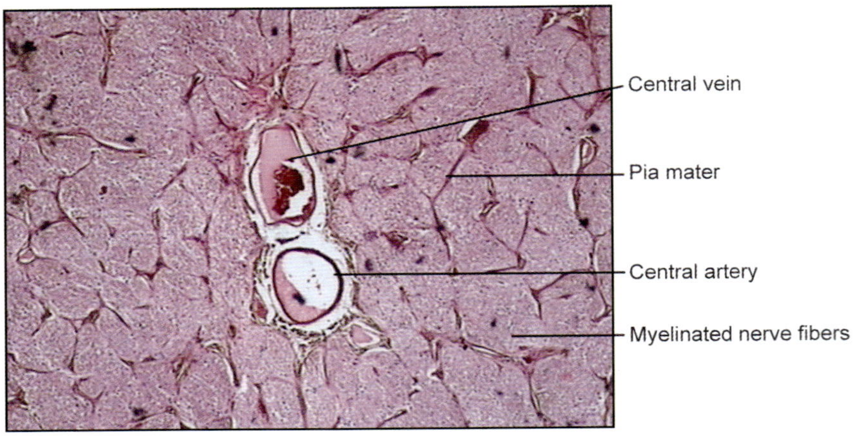

FIGURE 17.7 Optic nerve, H & E, X40

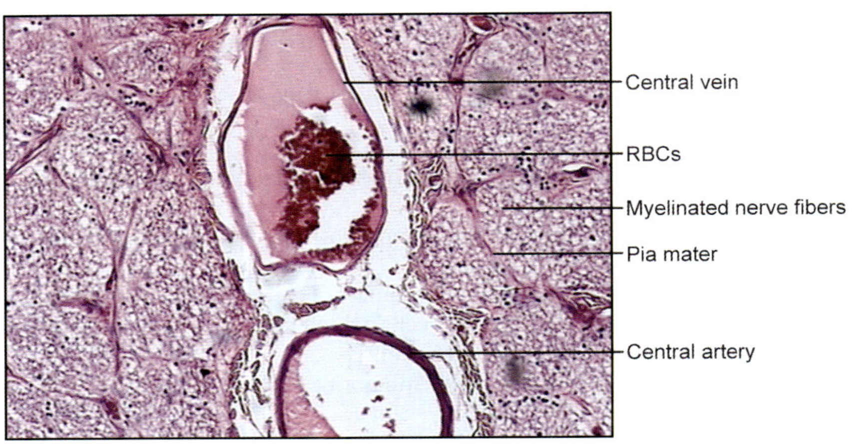

FIGURE 17.8 Optic nerve, H & E, X100

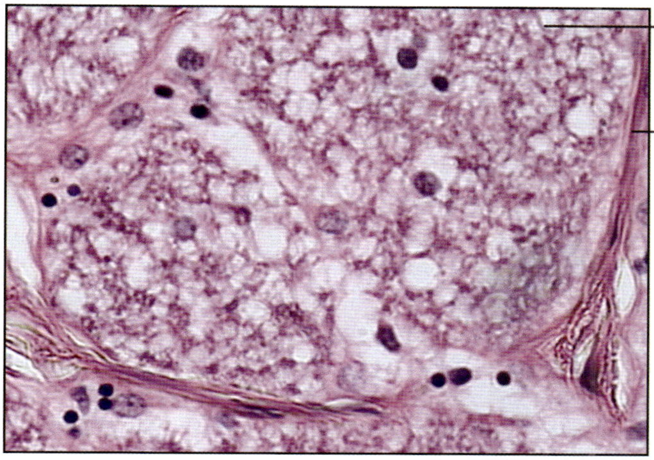

FIGURE 17.9 Optic nerve, H & E, X400

a delicate membrane made up of interlacing collagen fibers and fine elastic network covered by simple squamous epithelium. It sends in septa carrying the vasa nervosum within the optic nerve. It divides the optic nerve into several bundles of myelinated nerve fibers. The optic nerve contains a central artery and vein that traverse the lamina cribrosa. Branches of these blood vessels supply the inner portion of the retina. Central artery of retina courses through optic nerve and supplies blood to retina. The blood is drained from retina through capillary network and then to central vein of retina. The vessels supply optic nerve fiber layer of retina only, the superficial layers and peripheral layers are dependent on diffusion for the nutrition.

Sections under scanner (Fig. 17.7), low power (Fig. 17.8) and high power (Fig. 17.9) show the central artery and vein of retina surrounded by the bundles of the nerve fibers. The bundles of the nerve fibers are separated from each other by the septa formed by the pia mater. The nerve fibers present in the bundles are myelinated.

POINTS TO REMEMBER

Cornea

Corneal epithelium	Nonkeratinized stratified squamous epithelium Microvilli on the cell surface helps in retaining film of fluid over the corneal surface
Bowman's membrane	Homogeneous thin layer made of fine collagen fibrils
Substantia propria	Thickest layer, type 2 collagen fibers embedded in ground substance with sulphated glycosaminoglycans in the form of lamellae, transparency due to regular arrangement of fibers and cells
Descemet's membrane	Highly refractive homogeneous layer
Endothelium	Low cuboidal epithelium

Retina

Pigment layer	Single layer of hexagonal cells with pigment granules
Layer of rods and cones	Arranged parallel, perpendicular to the surface
External limiting membrane	Sieve-like membrane formed by Müller's fibers
Outer nuclear layer	Nuclei of rods and cones
Outer plexiform layer	Reticular meshwork formed by: Terminal fibers of rods and cones, the dendrites of bipolar cells
Inner nuclear layer	*Nuclei of:* Bipolar cells, horizontal cells, amacrine cells
Inner plexiform layer	*Processes of:* Amacrine cells, axons of bipolar cells, dendrites of ganglion cells
Ganglion cell layer	Multipolar ganglion cells, neuroglia cells, retinal blood vessels
Nerve fiber layer	Axons of ganglion cells between which are fibrous neuroglia cells, rows of Müller's fibers and retinal blood vessels
Internal limiting membrane	Expanded bases of Müller's cells

Optic Nerve

- Surrounded by outer dura mater, inner pia mater and intermediate arachnoid mater.
- Sheaths continuous with the corresponding meninges of the brain and at the bulb, continuous with the sclera.
- Groups of fiber bundles enclosed by the septa arise from the pia mater.
- Septa united to form the central supporting tissue strand in the anterior part of the nerve, about half inch behind the eye, carry the central artery and central vein of the retina, eccentric in position.

CHAPTER

18

Central Nervous System

INTRODUCTION

The central nervous system consists of brain and spinal cord. The brain and spinal cord, is very delicate and is protected by bones (skull, vertebrae), connective tissue layers (meninges) and watery cerebrospinal fluid (CSF).

The brain and spinal cord contain both gray matter and white matter. The gray matter consists of neurons, dendrites and supportive cells, the neuroglia and represents the site of synapses between neurons and dendrites. White matter is devoid of neurons and consists of myelinated axons.

Neurons are the structural and functional unit of nervous system being more than 10 billion. There are three types of neurons, the sensory, motor and interneurons. Sensory are unipolar, motor and interneurons are multipolar. Neurons do not divide, but in some regions neural stem cells are able to differentiate and replace the damaged nerve cells. Neuroglia is highly branched, supportive, non-neuronal cells located between the neurons. Neuroglia does not get stimulated or conduct impulses and they are morphologically and functionally different from the neurons. The cells are smaller in size and nuclei stain darkly. Neuroglial cells are ten fold more in number than neurons. The four types of neuroglia are the astrocytes, oligodendrocytes, microglia and ependymal cells.

SPINAL CORD

Basic structural pattern is seen throughout the spinal cord, but the shape and structure of the cord vary in different regions. The meninges dura mater, arachnoid mater and pia mater surround the spinal cord.

The spinal cord is divided into two halves by anterior median fissure and posterior median sulcus. The spinal cord has two parts, the outer white matter having ascending and descending nerve fibers, the inner gray matter having cell bodies as well as nerve fibers. The white matter is divided into anterior, lateral and posterior funiculi. The gray matter is H-shaped in structure with ventral horn (anterior gray column) and dorsal horn (posterior gray column). The ventral horn has motor neurons and the dorsal horn has neurons that receive information from sensory neurons located in the dorsal root ganglia. The lateral gray horns are seen in thoracic and upper part of lumbar parts only containing the motor neurons of sympathetic division of autonomic nervous system. The connection in the center between the two sides of gray matter is called gray commissure.

The size of the gray matter is different in different regions of the spinal cord. In the cervical region (Fig. 18.1) the spinal cord is compressed anteroposteriorly and oval in the lower cervical region. The white matter is greater than the gray matter. Thoracic part (Fig. 18.2) shows slender dorsal horns and smaller ventral horns with fewer motor neurons. The lateral horns are well-developed in the thoracic region. In the lumbar region (Fig. 18.3) the spinal cord is larger and oval. There is relatively little white matter and both columns of gray matter are very thick, but anterior

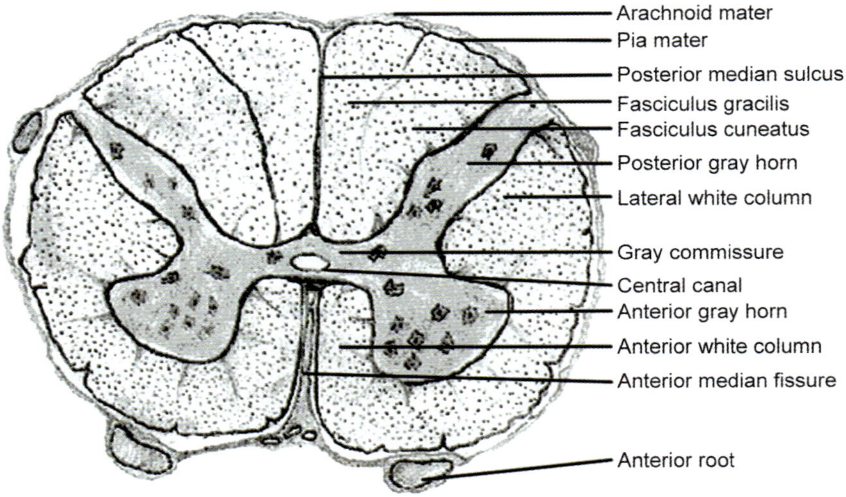

FIGURE 18.1 Spinal cord, cervical region, diagrammatic

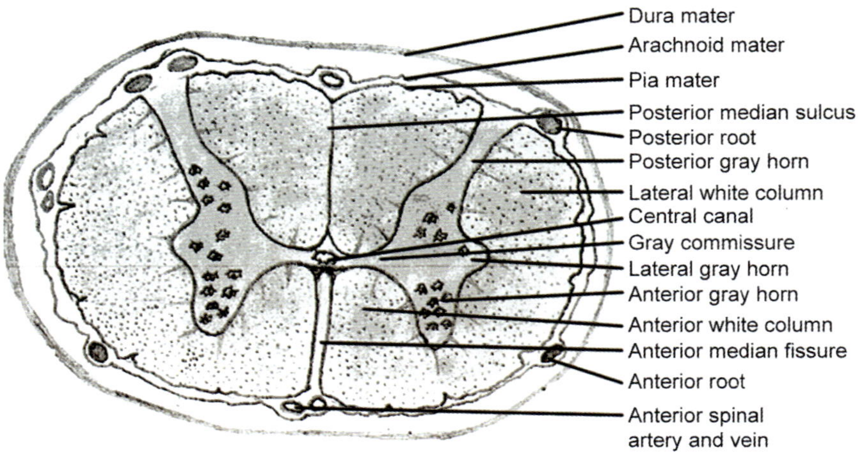

FIGURE 18.2 Spinal cord, thoracic region diagrammatic

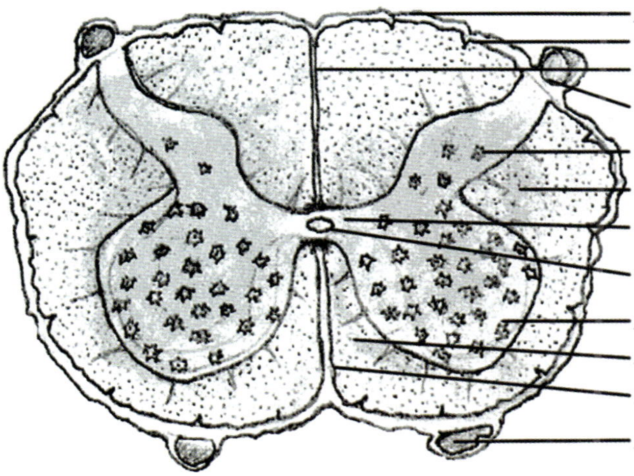

FIGURE 18.3 Spinal cord, lumbar region diagrammatic

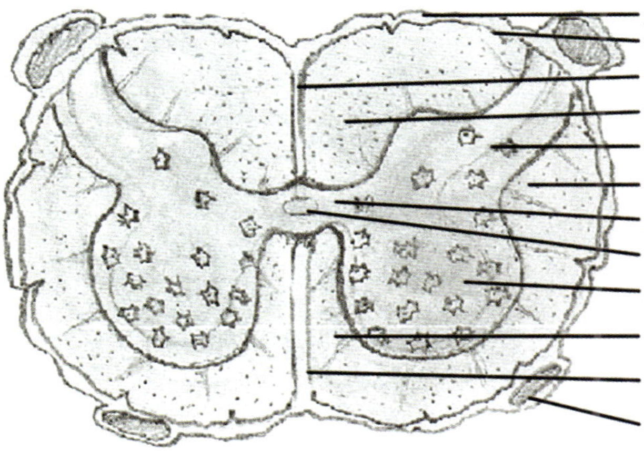

FIGURE 18.4 Spinal cord, sacral region diagrammatic

is thicker than posterior. In sacral region (Fig. 18.4) the spinal cord is very small in size. The white matter is very less compared to the gray matter. Both columns of gray matter are very thick.

CEREBRUM

Cerebrum is the main part of the brain that receives and stores the sensory information, control voluntary motor activity, integrate and coordinate the activity of other parts.

The section under scanner (Figs 18.5A and B) shows the gray matter of cerebrum that is present in the periphery. The white matter is present in the deep part of cerebrum is not seen in the photomicrograph. The whole thickness of the cerebrum is formed by gray matter, which forms the

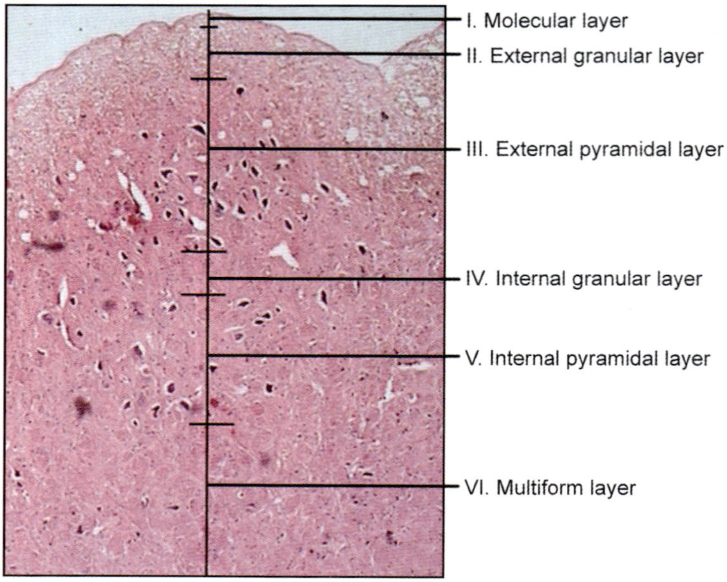

FIGURE 18.5A Cerebrum, H & E, X40

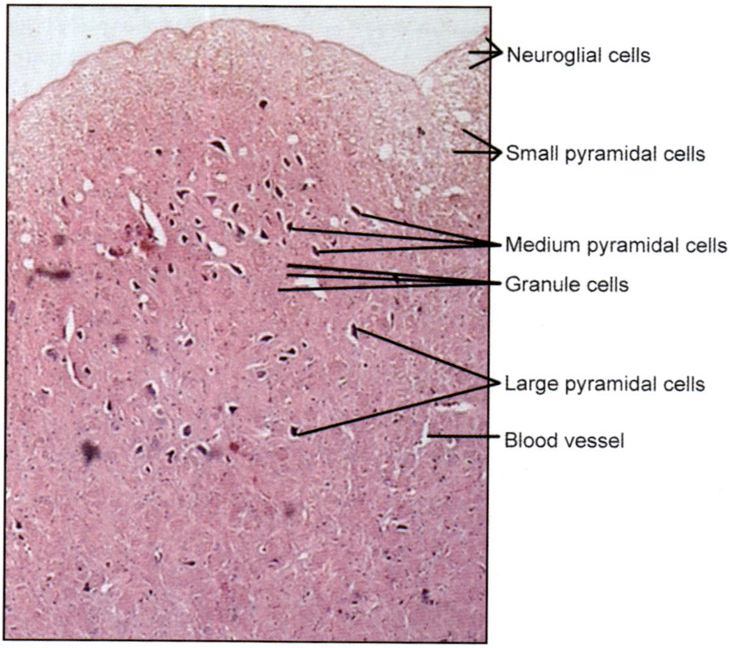

FIGURE 18.5B Cerebrum, H & E, X40

cortex of cerebrum. The cerebral cortex is covered by pia mater and is divided into six layers. Each layer is identified on the basis of predominant cell type and fiber arrangement.

1. *The plexiform layer or molecular layer:* It consists largely of fibers, most of which travel parallel to the surface and relatively few cells, mostly neuroglial cells and occasional horizontal cell of Cajal. The nuclei of neuroglial cells appear naked, since the cytoplasm is indistinguishable from nerve fibers.
2. The small pyramidal cell layer or outer granular layer. It consists mainly of small pyramidal cells and granule cells or stellate cells that are difficult to identify.
3. The layer of medium pyramidal cells or layer of outer pyramidal cells. It is not demarcated clearly from the second layer. It consists of medium-sized pyramidal cells that are larger in size.
4. *The granular layer or inner granular layer:* It consists of numerous small granule cells.
5. *The layer of large pyramidal cells or inner layer of pyramidal cells:* It consists of pyramidal cells that are smaller than the pyramidal cells in the third layer in many parts of the cerebrum, but in the motor area the pyramidal cells are extremely large and are called the Betz cells.
6. *The layer of polymorphic cells or multiform layer:* It consists of cells with diverse shapes many of which have spindle or fusiform shape. The cells are pyramidal cells, fusiform cells, granule cells and Martinotti cells.

CEREBELLUM

The cerebellum is part of the brain present behind and below cerebrum. It coordinates both voluntary movements and muscle function in the maintenance of normal posture.

The section under scanner (Fig. 18.6) shows the cortex and white matter of cerebellum. The gray matter present at the periphery form the cortex and white matter is present deep to the cortex. The cerebellar cortex shows deeply convoluted folds, the cerebellar folia separated by the sulci covered by the pia mater. Three layers are differentiated from outside, the outer molecular layer, middle Purkinje cell layer and inner granular layer. The molecular layer has few cells and horizontally directed fibers. The Purkinje cells are pyriform or pyramidal in shape with ramified dendrites that extend into molecular layer. Inner granular layer has small granule cells and large Golgi type II cells.

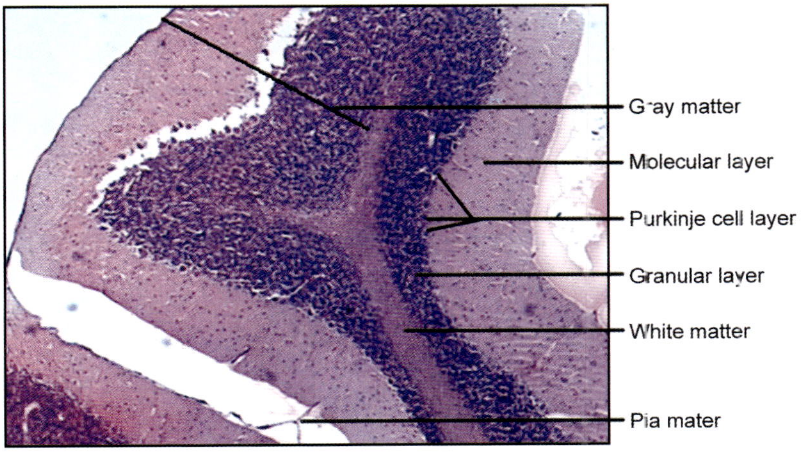

FIGURE 18.6 Cerebellum, H & E, X40

The white matter forms the core of each cerebellar folium consisting of myelinated nerve fibers that are afferent and efferent to cerebellar cortex.

The sections under low power (Fig. 18.7) and high power (Fig. 18.8) show the three layers of the cerebellum. The molecular layer consists of the scattered basket cells, the unmyelinated axons of which course normally in horizontal direction. Axons of the granule cells in granular layer extend into the molecular layer and also run horizontally as unmyelinated axons. The Purkinje cells in the Purkinje cell layer have prominent nuclei and nucleoli and are arranged in single layer at the junction of the molecular and granular layers. The cells have flask-shaped bodies and give off one or more thick dendrites that extend through the molecular layer to the surface and one thin axon from the base of the cell pass through the granular layer and reach the white matter. The granular layer has numerous small granule cells with dark staining nuclei and small amount of cytoplasm.

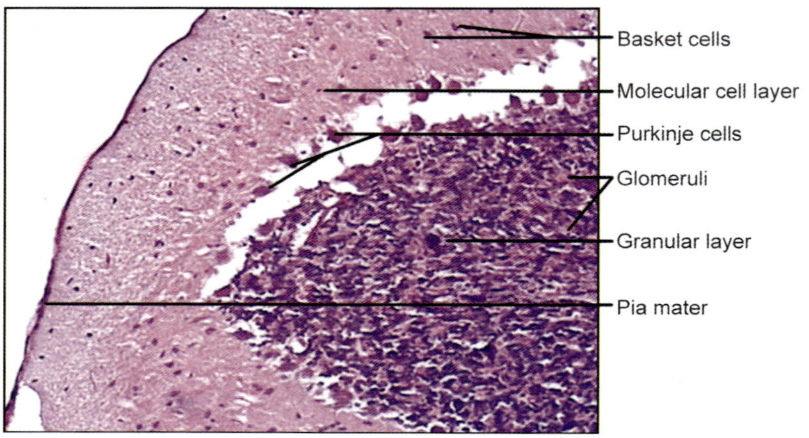

FIGURE 18.7 Cerebellum, H & E, X100

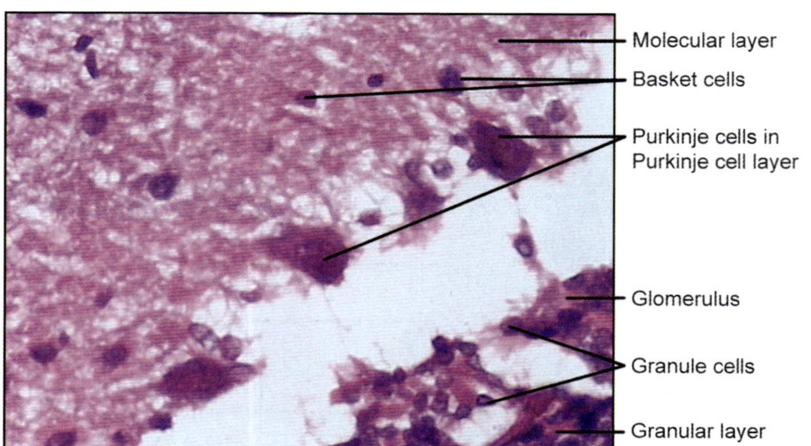

FIGURE 18.8 Cerebellum, H & E, X400

The Golgi type II cells are also present in between granule cells with typical vesicular nucleus and more cytoplasm. There are clear spaces called glomeruli scattered throughout granular layer containing synaptic complexes.

POINTS TO REMEMBER

Spinal Cord

The meninges, the dura mater, arachnoid mater and pia mater surround the spinal cord.

The spinal segments contributing to the nerves of upper limbs and lower limbs are enlarged to form the cervical and lumbar enlargements respectively.

The cross-sections in general consists of:

- White matter consisting of ascending and descending fibers is subdivided into anterior, lateral and posterior funiculi.
- Central gray matter consisting of nerve cells is divided into anterior gray column and posterior gray column.
- Central canal is in the middle of the gray matter.

The relative amount of gray and white matter and the shape and size of gray columns vary at different levels of spinal cord. The white matter increases from sacral to cervical levels of spinal cord.

	Cervical region	*Thoracic region*	*Lumbar region*
Shape	Compressed antero-posteriorly, oval in the lower cervical region	Rounded in outline and relatively small in size	Larger and oval
Composition	White matter greater than gray matter	Additional gray column, the lateral gray column, present on the lateral side between the anterior and posterior columns	Relatively little white matter; both columns of gray matter very thick, but anterior is more thick than posterior

Cerebrum

It has six layers or laminae from superficial surface downwards:

Plexiform or molecular layer	Predominantly fibers with few neuroglial cells, horizontal cells of Cajal
External granular layers	Predominantly stellate cells, small pyramidal cells
External pyramidal layer	Mainly pyramidal cells with some stellate cells, basket cells
Internal granular layer	Mainly closely arranged stellate cells, few pyramidal cells, interneurons, external band of Baillarger
Internal pyramidal layer or ganglionic layer	Giant pyramidal cells of Betz, internal band of Baillarger
Multiform or polymorphous layer	Fusiform cells, pyramidal cells, interneurons of various sizes and shapes

Difference between the granular and agranular cortex:

	Granular (sensory) cortex	*Agranular (motor) cortex*
Areas	Postcentral gyrus, visual cortex and acoustic areas	Precentral gyrus, area number 4, 6, 8, 44 and in parts of limbic system
Layers	Granular layers highly developed while the pyramidal and ganglionic layers are poorly developed or absent. In visual area the external band of Baillarger is prominent and forms a white line that can be seen with the naked eye when it is fresh	External and internal granular laminae are inconspicuous

Cerebellum

Structure is uniform in all parts of cerebellum.

Three layers from surface to the white matter.

Molecular layer	• Stellate and basket cells. • Mainly a synaptic zone, made up of profusely branching dendrites of Purkinje cells and the axons of granule cells.
Purkinje cell layer	• Layer named after the cells. • Single row of bodies of Purkinje cells.
Granular layer	• Granule cells and Golgi cells. • Axons of the cells extend into the molecular layer.

Bibliography

1. Antony L. Mescher. Junqueira's Basic Histology—Text and Atlas. 13th edn. Singapore: McGraw Hill, 2013.
2. Eroschenko. diFiore's Atlas of Histology with Functional Correlations. 11th edn. Indian edition reprint, New Delhi: BI Publications Pvt Ltd, 2009.
3. Susan Standring. Gray's Anatomy—The Anatomical Basis of Clinical Practice. 40th edn. Spain: Elsevier, 2008.
4. Ross MH, Pawlina W. Histology—A Text and Atlas with Correlated Cell and Molecular Biology. China: Lippincott Williams and Wilkins, 2011.
5. Singh IB. Textbook of Human Histology with Colour Atlas. 5th edn. New Delhi: Jaypee Brothers Medical Publishers (P) Ltd., 2006.
6. Young B, Lowe JS, Stevens A, Heath JW. Wheater's Functional Histology—A Text and Colour Atlas. New Delhi: Elsevier India Pvt Ltd., Indian reprint, 2007.

Index

Page numbers followed by *f* refer to figure

L

M

N

O

P

R